FEED YOUR PURPOSE

Intuitive Eating as a Spiritual Practice

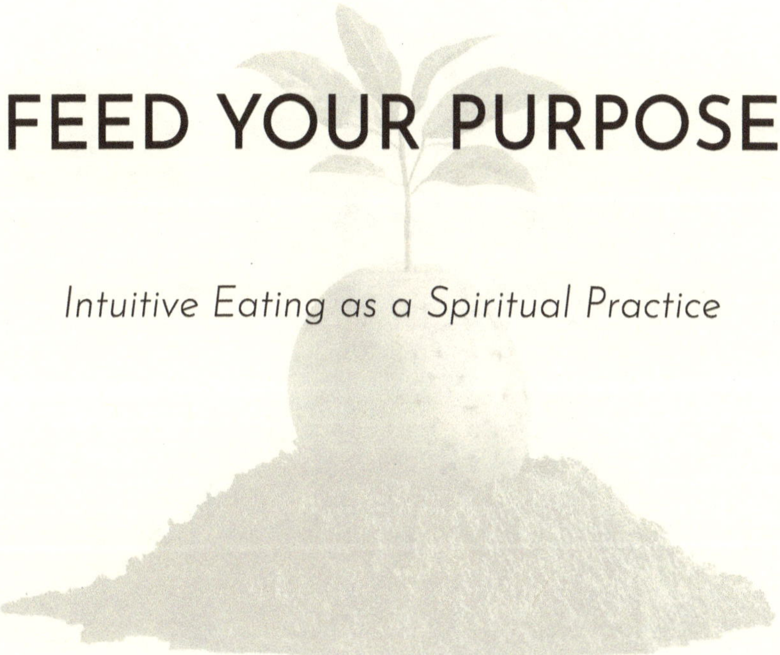

Sandi Morse, LCSW-S

Feed Your Purpose: Intuitive Eating as a Spiritual Practice

eBook: 979-8-234-00801-5
Paperback: 979-8-234-00802-2

For those learning to listen to their bodies
in a world that taught them not to, you are already whole.

For my soul dog Tarzan, who crossed the rainbow bridge as I wrote the conclusion of this book. Thank you for your unconditional love and the joy you brought to my life every day. I miss you deeply.

Disclaimer: This book is intended as a general guide and for informational purposes only. While I am a licensed clinician, I am not your personal clinician. This content should not replace professional, medical, or mental health advice tailored to your individual needs. Please take what serves you and know that support is out there when you need it. Resources for finding professional services are available at the end of the book.

Beyond a wholesome discipline,
be gentle with yourself.

You are a child of the universe,
no less than the trees and the stars;
you have a right to be here.
And whether or not it is clear to you,
no doubt the universe is unfolding as it should.

Therefore be at peace with God,
whatever you conceive Him to be,
and whatever your labors and aspirations,
in the noisy confusion of life keep peace with your soul.

With all its sham, drudgery, and broken dreams,
it is still a beautiful world.
Be cheerful.
Strive to be happy.

— "Desiderata," Max Ehrmann, 1927

TABLE OF CONTENTS

Chapter One

The Universe Has Better Plans for You

She sat on the edge of the small couch in my office with her arms crossed tightly around a throw pillow covering her stomach. She looked at me sadly and said, almost apologetically, "I'm so tired of feeling like this. I obsess about food. I've literally tried every diet, and I still hate my body. It's so depressing. I don't know why I'm like this." I had heard this story hundreds of times before. Different ages, different genders, different bodies, different details, but always the same shame. Always the same belief that something was wrong with them rather than with the system.

Do you remember the moment you started spending more time counting the number of calories you ate instead of the number of stuffed animals on your bed? Or the number of baseball cards in your collection? Can you recall the first time you declined a summer pool party because it would require you to be seen in a swimsuit? Do you remember peddling so fast on your bike in your neighborhood trying to race home before curfew, working up a sweat but with zero thoughts of calories being burned? When did your focus shift from having a wildly adventurous life to having a life hemmed in by worrying about counting calories, macros, and steps? **When was the last time your mind felt so free and full of love and hope that there was no space for thoughts of self-criticism?** That was the golden age of innocence, when anything and everything was possible, and we were going to do it all.

So how did we become entrenched in self-defeating cycles that keep us restricting our food intake, feeling guilty for eating a cookie, and running on the hamster wheel of dieting, losing, and regaining the same pounds every year? Why do we value other's opinions about our body shapes and sizes over our own opinions about ourselves? Why do we allow society to tell us what's an acceptable weight? If you've ever asked yourself these or similar questions or have grown angry towards yourself for what may feel like years of wasted time, you're in good company.

I think we can agree that early humans didn't start out counting macros and worrying about their animal skin clothing getting too tight. It was quite the opposite. They were worried about finding the next meal. They didn't cut the excess fat off their saber-toothed tiger steaks. They needed the calories to survive! But times have definitely changed, and we certainly didn't get here overnight. When did this obsession with how we eat and the size and shape of our bodies begin?

The earliest known diet in recorded history dates back to ancient Egypt, around 1500 BCE, and included diet regimens to treat various health conditions. But it's an English undertaker named William Banting (not a medical professional) who is credited with the first diet for the purposes of weight loss back in 1863, which was essentially a low-carb diet. This also set in motion the first example we have of someone using their own personal experience for public recommendations when it comes to diet, something we will see time and time again since. His case marked the birth of the modern self-help, weight-loss movement.

As Banting was touting the health benefits of going low-carb, across the Atlantic in the 1840s, Sylvester Graham (yes, graham crackers), an American Presbyterian minister, was preaching about the moral benefits of abstaining from spices, stimulants, and over-indulgences, all of which he attributed to sexual promiscuity, unrest, and more. While Pastor Graham wasn't the first to connect morality with dieting, his specific brand of dieting unfortunately became quite popular.

Since then, there has been no shortage of diets marketed to the masses. At the time of this publication, there are upwards of thirty mainstream diets all promising the same two things: one, their diet is different from all the others, and two, theirs is the only one that works.

If you're feeling skeptical, you're right to feel that way. The truth is, research shows that only 5 percent of diets work. The statistic that "95 percent of diets fail" is widely cited in discussions about weight loss, though the exact figure varies depending on the study and methodology. Yet, 100 percent of us truly believe we will be in that 5 percent. As you can see, the math doesn't add up. So how do so many of us fall into this trap? How is it possible that so many of us are not only duped into believing we'll be in the 5 percent but then blame ourselves when we're not?

Enter the weight loss product industry. Worth over $73 billion in the US alone—that's right, *billion*—this industry is dedicated to selling you a *product*. They have brilliant marketing teams brainstorming all the different ways they can convince us that they care about our health ("it's not a diet, it's a lifestyle"). But as the former CFO of Weight Watchers shared with the public, the truth is that the company's number one source of revenue is repeat customers, and they're not the only ones hoping you "fail."

It's really a genius marketing ploy that works time after time after time:

- Convince the prospective customer that they need to lose weight.
- Convince the customer their company has the right product for the job.
- Convince the customer it's simple and easy and if the product isn't working, it's the customer's fault.
- When the product fails, convince the customer to try again, and this time try harder. And again. And again.

Like I said, it's genius. Can you think of any other product that if it failed 95 percent of the time, they would get away with blaming the customer? That's exactly what happens. Let that sink in. However, the research is clear that **genetics play a role in our shape and size, with some studies indicating that our genes have a significant 70 percent role.** This suggests that body weight is largely heritable. Yet we are still convinced that we didn't lose weight because somehow we didn't try hard enough. We didn't have enough willpower. There's something wrong with us. It couldn't be the diet.

Enter shame. Enter guilt. Enter self-criticism, and self-loathing. And so what do we do? We try again. Maybe it's a different weight loss product this time. Maybe this one will work. And inevitably when it doesn't work, around and around we go. But it is not your fault for falling into a trap that was set for you.

Perhaps you're thinking, *But it's not true! I did lose weight that one time* or *My coworker Sally Sue has been doing the (fill in the blank diet) and has lost X amount of pounds!* This is where it's important to define what success/failure means when it comes to a diet. Here are some hard truths coming your way so I hope you're sitting down.

There is little research that demonstrates sustained weight loss six months after dieting. There is, however, research that demonstrates that one-third of people who lose weight *will* gain it back. And one-third of those will gain *more* than they lost. A comprehensive review of thirty-one long-term, doctor-administered diet studies published in *American Psychologist* in 2007 found that approximately two-thirds of participants regained more weight than they had lost within four to five years. Similarly, a 2013 guideline from Australia's National Health and Medical Research Council (NHMRC) stated that most weight lost through dieting is regained within two years, and by five years, most individuals return to their original weight.

The number one predictor of weight gain? Dieting. Harsh, I know.

If you're done with dieting, if you're tired of letting others tell you what's acceptable about your body, if you're searching for a way to reconnect with self, if you want to heal from dieting trauma, keep reading. This is not a diet book. I will not tell you what to do while simultaneously offering false promises. This is not *The Seven Steps to Making Yourself Good Enough in Thirty Days!* Instead, this book aims to save you from all of the unnecessary and burdensome rules you've likely created for yourself around food, weight, and the size and shape of your body. This book will also help you repair your relationship with food, returning it to its original and simple purposes of fuel and pleasure, thus freeing your mind from all the noise and creating the much needed brainspace for what really matters: our connection to our faith and each other.

The Intersection of Food and Faith

The first time I heard the term *intuitive eating,* I was running an eating disorder clinic for women in Dallas in 2013. I'd had some prior exposure to working with eating disorders, but most of my clinical and administrative experience had been in general mental health and substance abuse. When I found myself immersed in the world of eating disorder treatment, I quickly learned that it has its own set of particular skills, therapeutic models, and processes that make it unique and extremely challenging. It requires addressing not only complex psychological and emotional issues but also deeply ingrained societal norms and trauma histories, not to mention very real, and sometimes very scary, medical concerns. Specialists must navigate a delicate balance between empathy and accountability while often working with clients who are ambivalent about recovery. Additionally, the lack of adequate training in graduate programs, limited professional support, and the emotional toll of witnessing clients with this level of severity can lead to burnout and compassion fatigue. It's no wonder why so few clinicians specialize in this work—it's really, really hard. According to Project Heal, fewer than 1 percent of mental health professionals specialize in eating disorders.

Fortunately, there are some places that just do it right. Working at that clinic was the best job I've ever had. Not only did I work with some of the most brilliant clinicians I've ever known that I am proud to say have transitioned from my colleagues to my friends, this experience also started me on my path in this space. Had I not worked in this specialty, I don't know that I ever would have learned about diet culture and anti-fat bias and intuitive eating.

Elyse Resch and Evelyn Tribole, two masters-level dieticians, are the founders and pioneers of intuitive eating. They were tired of preaching the status quo of a (slim) weight-focused health paradigm that consistently seemed to do more harm than good both psychologically and physically to the people they were trying to help. This led them to recognize and reconnect with the wisdom of the body, among other tenets, which they wrote about in their book *Intuitive Eating: A Revolutionary Diet Approach*. Originally published in 1995 and now in its fourth edition, it is a must read. As of this writing, it has sold over 500,000 copies, and the duo has developed an Intuitive Eating Counseling certification course for fellow dieticians and other clinicians. In fact, I am honored to say I have completed it myself.

In their book, Resch and Tribole describe intuitive eating as "a flexible style of eating in which you largely follow your internal sensations of hunger and satiety to gauge when to eat, what to eat, and when to stop eating." It's further defined as "a self-care eating framework that integrates instinct, emotion and rational thought…in a weight inclusive, evidence-based model, with a validated assessment scale and over 125 studies to date." The framework consists of ten principles:

- Principle One: Reject diet culture
- Principle Two: Honor your hunger
- Principle Three: Make peace with food
- Principle Four: Discover the satisfaction factor
- Principle Five: Feel your fullness
- Principle Six: Challenge the food police
- Principle Seven: Cope with your emotions with kindness
- Principle Eight: Respect your body
- Principle Nine: Movement—feel the difference
- Principle Ten: Honor your health—gentle nutrition

While the principles are numbered here, only the first one, "reject diet culture," and the last one, "honor your health—gentle nutrition," should be practiced in a specific order. So for the sake of this book, I chose this particular order that is in line with the order from the original founders of intuitive eating, but you can read them and practice them however you choose.

Each principle is designed to help people let go of the dysfunctional cultural obsession with thinness and the never-ending cycle of dieting and get back to a loving relationship with their bodies. After all, we didn't come out of the womb counting the calories in our bottles or our mother's milk. We were born to grow and learn, explore and connect, and love.

Most people find intuitive eating after having been in the vicious cycle of diet culture for most of their lives. By the time they get here, they are desperate for something different, and intuitive eating is definitely different. It doesn't come with any rules; instead, it asks you to trust that you are unique, and therefore, so are the ways that you need to honor your health and well-being. It's not the easiest path. For some, it will seem so natural that it feels like a tremendous relief. But for others, it will feel (and may be) a complete departure from everything they think they've known about nutrition, food, weight, and overall health, and this may feel scary or generate feelings of disbelief. After all, the model encourages you to let go of control and deeply held beliefs.

As John Steinbeck writes in his brilliant book *East of Eden,* "And this I believe: that the free, exploring mind of the individual human is the most valuable thing in the world. And this I would fight for: the freedom of the mind to take any direction it wishes, undirected." If you're new to intuitive eating, you are about to experience freedom in your own mind in a way you've probably never felt before. Even if you're an expert intuitive eater already, this book will help you take it to the next level and deepen your experiences with your faith and your relationships.

Before we go further, let's chat a bit about the word "intuitive." In her book *FulFilled,* Dr. Anna Yusim reminds us that intuition comes from the Latin *intuir,* which means "knowledge from within. . . . It is a subjective mental experience that gives us information about the present moment by enabling us to tap into our true self. . . . This inner voice exists within all of us; it has always been there and is actually communicating with us all the time."

She goes on to say, "Many believe that learning to hear one's inner voice and cultivating one's intuition is synonymous with connecting to one's soul." This is one of the many reasons why I believe intuitive eating and spirituality are complementary.

When we listen to our inner voice—whether it's related to our hunger cues or a gut check for a big decision or we're tuning into our emotions with silent reflection—it all comes from the same place, which is within ourselves. For some, this could mean tapping into the Holy Spirit or praying and listening for an answer from the Universe or their deity. This practice of turning inward may feel challenging or even daunting, especially if you've been caught up in diet culture. **Diet culture teaches us to ignore our internal wisdom and that our bodies don't know what they need.** It teaches us that our bodies must be controlled in some way because our natural way of being isn't good enough. Diet culture disconnects us from ourselves and causes us to be distrustful of our own bodies. But rest assured, turning inward is a skill that can be cultivated, and the reward is worth it.

More than that, though, I've found that when we cultivate this intuition in conjunction with our faith and reactivate the intrinsic bond between the two, both become a strong, almost unstoppable force for our well-being. After all, an estimated 90 percent of people believe in some kind of higher power, and more than 70 percent of people identify their faith or spirituality as important in their lives. Why wouldn't you include your faith and spirituality as guidance in decisions you make about your body?

Before we continue, a side note about faith and belief systems: Faith is a personal and unique experience. When I say *faith* in this book, I'm simply referring to the idea that there is something bigger than ourselves and our individual human experience, whatever religion or deities you follow. If you look closely, you find there are universal truths that multiple different faiths and religions of the world have in common. Simply put, faith is trust or confidence in someone or something in the context of religion or spirituality. For me, right now, that means God.

For most of my life, I've vacillated between identifying myself as religious or spiritual, even in times when I was practicing neither. I grew up in a strict Catholic church but later realized that some of the teachings no longer aligned with my beliefs, so I stopped attending services. Shortly after this, during my yoga certification and for many years thereafter, I became very involved with both Hindu and Buddhist religions and the concept of spirituality as a whole. Later in life, as a result of my peer group at the time, I found my way to a progressive Methodist church, which is where I currently practice my faith.

I sincerely believe that everyone will find value in the chapters of this book, including my agnostic and atheist readers. It's fair to say that I frame it through my God lens; however, I've strived to be as inclusive as possible. It is because of my faith that I believe God loves us and that our big, bold purpose in life is to love one another, not to worry about our size.

Our preoccupations with food and weight are holding us back from our higher purpose. I can promise you that **our purpose is not to shrink our bodies into being as small as possible.** I believe that God and the Universe want so much more for us and how we spend the precious little time we have. The noise around diets and macros and calories and step counts and rules and restrictions and what to eat and what not to eat and the never-ending pursuit of weight loss is all consuming for many. I believe that letting it go frees up invaluable mental real estate. I believe that God and the Universe are ready to rush in and fill that space up with a higher calling.

Seeking Something More

I believe that most, if not all, of us are seekers. We're trying to live lives that feel connected and worth living. We're yearning for a sense of purpose and meaning, yet the majority of our days are wrapped up in the business of life. We begin to feel lost, as if we're on autopilot and always spinning our wheels. As a licensed clinical social worker, in both my lived and professional experience, the focus on our outer bodies instead of the souls we carry is what gets in the way and is the most insidious drain on our lives. If we truly are spiritual beings having a human experience, why waste one more second not enjoying that experience? Why waste one more breath asking how many grams of fat are in that salad dressing?

If you are searching for a way that truly honors both your physical and mental health, then intuitive eating is your best chance for success. In a 2018 meta-analysis of intuitive eating studies, researchers found that intuitive eating enhanced body image, self-esteem, mental well-being, and quality of life while decreasing depression, anxiety, body dissatisfaction, and negative self-talk. This intuitive eating path, paved with truth and self-compassion, is free from the roadblocks of misinformation, shame, and guilt. It will bring you to a better relationship with food and your body than you ever thought was possible. And it will give you the mental space you need to ponder the big questions in life.

There is a path to a greater connection with your life's purpose after you've been unburdened of all the noise in your head about how, what, when, where, and why we eat along with all of the conditioned judgment and guilt you're "supposed" to feel about eating.

Throughout the rest of this book, we will explore the ten principles of intuitive eating. Each chapter will deep-dive into one of the ten principles, investigating why and how diet culture has convinced us we're not already the perfectly-made beings we are, along with the spiritual teachings that clearly demonstrate you were meant for something more than counting calories or food points or worrying about what number is on the tag inside clothes. Finally, every chapter will end with an exercise or two that aims to help you rebuild trust with your inherent body wisdom.

In writing this book, I didn't want to rely only upon my personal experience—too many books do that already. So I draw from both research and the lived experiences of people from many different walks of life. As such, I have included perspectives and interviews with individuals from varying religious and spiritual backgrounds.

Whether you are a devout practitioner of your identified religious belief or consider yourself a spiritual seeker and are open to and fascinated by the questions of purpose, meaning, our Universe, and how the spiritual intersects with food, you are no doubt a child of the Universe who deserves a better life than diet culture would have you live. You are not broken. You do not need fixing. You do not need to "slim down" to be acceptable and be accepted. You are perfect right now. And you deserve all of the joy and happiness and fulfillment of living a life of deep connection with God and the Universe and chocolate cake. Interested? Wonderful. Let's get started.

Chapter Two

Reject Diet Culture and Let Go of False Promises

As Julie Andrews would say, " Let's start at the very beginning. A very good place to start." I wish I could say that the principles start out easy and get increasingly difficult as you become more comfortable with the philosophy of intuitive eating, but my experience and the experiences of my former patients have been that the first principle is the hardest. Before you are even taught any of the brilliant skills (and they are brilliant), you must first decide that you've had enough.

In Chapter 1, we touched on the structure of diet culture and how it mentally and emotionally affects us, the would-be consumers. Here's the biggest takeaway: Diet culture does not exist to help anyone. It is an industry that exists to make money. Period.

You don't want to keep feeling badly about yourself. Your body and your mind are tired of being obsessed with food and the scale and all the noise from all the diets you've tried over the years. Coming to these conclusions isn't that difficult. If you picked up this book, I would suspect you're already there. But what is harder (much, much harder) is to make the decision that you will not try another diet.

Rejecting diet culture means that when the next new shiny weight-loss product is released (and as sure as I'm writing this, another one will be released this year), you will not fall for the false promises wrapped up in brilliant marketing terminology. You will be able to say, even with shaky confidence, that you will not put your physical and mental health in jeopardy. You will invest your time, commitments, energy, and financial resources elsewhere. And you will give up on intentional weight loss because you have accepted your own biology.

Phew, what a leap, huh?

Because it can feel daunting to let go of a system that may have subtly and not so subtly directed your life and choices for far too long, this chapter is quite robust. Not only are we speaking about current diet culture and how it controls us, we are also discussing its deep historical roots. Nothing springs up overnight, especially not a $73 billion industry. It's my hope to break down the complex web of research, science, history, and cultural context to make this easy for you. As I've already said and will say again, you deserve more than a sugar-free imitation of life.

Now let's talk about what diet culture actually entails.

What We Mean When We Say "Diet Culture"

Diet culture is an oppressive system of beliefs that not only idealizes thinness but erroneously equates thinness with health, resulting in a continuous cycle of dieting in pursuit of weight loss to achieve the thin ideal. Diet culture is the never-ending, unrelenting, self-sabotaging, uphill battle of achieving a specific ideal body type that changes with the decade and will be unattainable for the vast majority of people.

Diet culture is sneaky. It hides in the rebranded marketing,

"It's not a diet; it's a lifestyle." It's in the endless obsessive counting of calories, macros, and steps. It's in concepts like "cheat days." It's in unnecessary and unresearched detoxes and cleanses. It's in the heartbreaking and perpetual sense of failure so many of us feel because, despite our success in other areas of life, we still don't have the bodies we had at 25, even though we're now 45. It underlies the statement "I just want to be healthy," when what that really means is "I want to be thin."

Now let me be clear. Rejecting diet culture does not mean people don't want to be healthy, nor am I saying that. Of course they do. We all do. What I'm saying is that you can be healthy and live in a larger body, even though diet culture has led us to believe otherwise and convinced us that this isn't what people truly want.

Diet culture is the reason that, for so many of us, the size and shape of our bodies is directly tied to our sense of self-worth. Combine this with a lack of prioritizing our connection to our faith and spirituality, and it creates this fascinating and incredibly harmful distortion that we're not innately worthy, but rather, our worth is directly connected to our appearance. Diet culture is the wildly inaccurate belief that none of our accomplishments, talents, and positive qualities amounts to anything if we aren't also the ideal (read "thin") body type. Diet culture tells us all of these falsehoods instead of the truth, which is that **the mere existence of our unique, one-of-a-kind selves, with zero replication in the Universe, is an absolute miracle.** And yet, diet culture's noise is so loud, it overpowers what we know deep down to be true and instead focuses on our appearance as the ultimate evidence of worth.

What's additionally fascinating and still incredibly harmful is how accepted and normalized this has become in our society. We don't question diet culture's unearned authority on the matter, and we often skip over the spiritual implications of what it means to give diet culture that authority. **When we allow diet culture to determine our worth, we cut out any higher power or spiritual**

design that created us. Because really, wouldn't that higher power have the right to the final say? Instead, we give that power to others who do not have our best interest in their hearts.

Taking it further, **diet culture has focused our attention so much on physical appearance that it's created a divide between body and spirit.** We no longer consider that maybe our body was perfectly designed to be a certain way. Rather, we think we've failed to control our eating habits. We've completely removed God from the equation. In fact, my friend shared with me that in all of her years as a pastor, she's never had anyone come to her with concerns about body image struggles. She's probably ministered to thousands of people in her life. Does that mean none of them had any body image struggles? Of course not. What we can infer is that oftentimes individuals may not seek out spiritual advisors with body image concerns because we've normalized those concerns. We've completely forgotten that God gave us this body for a purpose and with a purpose. We're meant for so much more, but diet culture has stolen that "more" from us.

The Problems with How We Measure "Health"

Without diet culture dictating how we should look and what we should eat, what do we do? We've been told by everyone for all of our lives that thin equals healthy. So we have to keep trying to lose weight, right? Well, let's unpack that.

Imagine that you are attending a social event and getting to know some new people. A mutual friend introduces you to two women you've never met. First is Veronica, a woman who has a larger body type that might be described as "heavy," and then there's Anne, a woman with a small body type that might be described as "slim." Your brain might automatically assume that Anne is healthier than Veronica. Diet culture has conditioned us to believe this.

First (and if you take nothing else from this book, please remember this), you *cannot* tell the health of any individual based on their size. Research supports that weight is a poor indicator of health. There are people who are in smaller bodies who are unhealthy, and people in larger bodies who are perfectly healthy. Full stop.

Skeptical? Now it's time to tell you more about Anne and Veronica.

Anne works in computer engineering. She spends nearly all of her time in front of the computer in a windowless room with her coworkers until they head to the local bar after work, where she drinks beer and smokes the occasional cigarette. She has a ton of deadlines, and if she remembers to eat at all, it's usually from the vending machine in the hall at work. She is anxious, stressed, and only getting four hours of sleep a night. Remember that Anne is in a small body.

Veronica works in a hair salon. She spends all day on her feet but loves her job and her customers. She spends most of the day laughing. After work she comes home and makes a meal with her spouse. They love to try new recipes. Each evening after their meal, they walk their dogs around the neighborhood. She gets a full eight hours of quality sleep every night. Remember that Veronica is in a large body.

Now, which of these two women do you believe is likely the healthier of the two? My guess is you would select Veronica. But would you have selected her before knowing the background if she was just standing side by side with Anne?

There are millions of examples we could use to illustrate the point, and I hope this offers a different perspective. This is also why **before-and-after pictures can be misleading and even harmful. Show me the before-and-after bloodwork**, and maybe I'll be more convinced. But the sad truth is that we have been conditioned to believe larger bodies are unhealthy and that the only way to be healthy is to shrink ourselves into a smaller body. And the only way to do that? You guessed it—a weight-loss product. However, that kind of thinking doesn't benefit us; it benefits the weight-loss company's bottom line.

Perhaps you're thinking, *Okay, Sandi, I hear you, but I know I'm still overweight.* My response: "Over what weight?" What is your benchmark? Is it the Body Mass Index, often referred to as BMI? If that's the case, here's a short history lesson.

Once upon a time, almost two hundred years ago, there lived a Belgian astronomer and mathematician named Adolphe Quetelet. Adolphe, who was interested in the statistics of the "average man" and the population at large, very much wanted to make a name for himself and his country in academia. He began gathering any data he could get his hands on, one of the data sets being height and weight charts. Eventually he published his work and called it the Quetelet Index. He wanted his work to help assess population trends, not be used for clinical use or to assess individual health.

An important note here is that Adolphe was specifically interested in the average *European* man. As such, his sample size came from mostly French and Scottish soldiers and was not representative of women or people of color. Over time, many people liked Adolphe's data sets and accompanying easy-to-use formulas as a measure of "health." Then, in the 1970s, psychologist and dietician Ancel Keys promoted the Quetelet Index as the best way to determine obesity, and the Body Mass Index entered mainstream clinical practice.

In the 1990s, the World Health Organization (WHO) changed the BMI categories based on recommendations from the International Obesity Task Force. Overnight, people moved into higher BMI categories because the WHO had changed the groupings. It's important to note that pharmaceutical companies funded almost the entirety of the International Obesity Task Force. At this point, it's clear who benefits from using faulty data to move millions of Americans into higher BMI weight categories, and, therefore, higher risk categories. And that's not even touching the conflict of interest issues.

If you've ever been on the receiving end of being told your BMI is anything but "normal," you may have experienced a sense of shame or guilt about this and/or been made to feel shameful or guilty. And yet, many health care providers agree the BMI is at best flawed, and at worst, harmful in its use for individual health purposes. In fact, a 2008 study in the Archives of Internal Medicine found that relying on BMI resulted in misclassification of healthy versus unhealthy. Specifically, the study reported that 51.3 percent of "overweight" and 31.7 percent of "obese" individuals were metabolically healthy, whereas 23.5 percent of "normal" weight individuals had at least two cardiometabolic abnormalities.

In 2016, UCLA took this a step further when it published a study analyzing data from the 2005-2012 National Health and Nutrition Examination Survey (NHANES) that found 54 million Americans with an "overweight" or "obese" BMI designation were actually metabolically healthy when assessed using *other* health indicators, such as blood pressure, cholesterol, and glucose levels. Conversely, some individuals with a "normal" BMI were found to be metabolically unhealthy.

If you want to throw this book across the room, I get it. I'm deeply frustrated, too. Throw it and then come back because we are far from done.

Ready?

So the next natural question is why do so many doctors and clinicians still use the BMI?

The BMI has become so ingrained in our healthcare system that even if you go in for an ear infection, the med tech will likely weigh you first. Further, in many healthcare systems, like the one where my own physicians practice, the electronic medical record requires the chart document BMI, so even when I politely say, "No, thank you," to being weighed, they have to enter something. And so they continue to enter my weight from ten years ago, which is the last weight they have for me in their system. I'm rarely asked about it these days, fortunately, but every now and then, I'm asked why I don't want to be weighed. My mood usually predicts my response. Sometimes I'll reply with, "If you're willing to enter in my weight from ten years ago as part of my present health visit today, that should indicate how benign the metric really is in my overall health." But most of the time if asked, I'll just say, "If my doctor determines it's medically necessary, I'll be happy to hop on the scale." Honestly, I've only really received pushback a couple of times in my life. I imagine that if I lived in a larger body, the reaction to declining to be weighed would be very different.

Even still, I believe that the vast majority of health care providers care deeply about their patients and their profession and want to do the right thing by their patients. Yet the truth is that there is a very real medical bias against people in larger bodies. As such, this creates health inequity. People in larger bodies are less likely to go to the doctor due to fear of being mistreated or condescended to at the office. People in larger bodies are less likely to be referred to specialists and more likely to be labeled as non-compliant.

Hold on because it gets worse. People in larger bodies are sent for less diagnostic testing, resulting in misdiagnosis because symptoms are attributed to their weight *without proper screenings*. In fact, many providers and payor sources have BMI thresholds that allow them to deny coverage for surgeries and even fertility treatment until a patient loses weight to satisfy these arbitrary lists. They are often excluded from clinical trials and therefore not represented in the data and subsequent findings.

There are heartbreaking stories of patients who went to see their doctor with pain and symptoms only to be told they simply needed to lose weight when their conditions were quite serious. One way to challenge this biased treatment is to ask the provider, "What would you recommend if I were in a thinner body?" But that shouldn't be necessary. We all have biases, but medical providers have an ethical responsibility to check theirs at the door and treat all of their patients with dignity, respect, and the best possible care.

Some good news? Many weight-inclusive medical providers have started taking the stance that not only are weight and the BMI inadequate health measures, but that weight should primarily be used to determine medication and anesthesia dosages, and for certain medical equipment, such as a blood pressure cuff.

Change Is Coming, Slowly

In 2003, several clinicians and activists from various advocacy groups came together to found the Association for Size Diversity and Health (ASDAH). The organization's goal is to shift the focus from weight to well-being and to combine activism with academic research. The ASDAH is dedicated to educating the general population and medical community about medical anti-fat bias and advocating for healthcare to align with the Health at Every Size® (HAES) approach. It also promotes health behaviors without stigmatizing people based on body size and aims to create a more inclusive and compassionate approach to healthcare.

HAES has five core principles:

1. Weight inclusivity emphasizes that health and self-worth are not determined by body size.

2. Health enhancement supports equal access to care and health practices that improve well-being for everyone.

3. Respectful care calls for the end of weight bias in healthcare and recognizes the impact of social conditions on health.

4. Eating for well-being encourages flexible, intuitive eating guided by hunger, fullness, and enjoyment.

5. Life-enhancing movement promotes physical activity that is enjoyable and accessible to all, regardless of size or ability.

The work of ASDAH and the principles of HAES are well known to clinicians who work in the intuitive eating space. These ideals are slowly becoming more mainstream, but there is still so much work to be done.

If you were in the U.S. in the late 1990s and early 2000s, you couldn't turn on the news or look at a *Time* magazine cover without hearing or seeing something about the "obesity epidemic." Remember the WHO and the International Obesity Task Force and their terrible decisions regarding BMI? Well, in 1997, the WHO also popularized the term "obesity epidemic" to signify a public health crisis due to the *association* (not causation) between obesity and numerous chronic health conditions like type 2 diabetes, heart disease, and certain cancers. However, in 2013, the American Medical Association Council on Science and Public Health (CSAPH) recommended against classifying obesity as a disease after the committee shared its year-long review of the issue. The committee found that the BMI is an imperfect measure (duh), and that traditional diseases have a specific set of symptoms, whereas obesity does not, and that outcomes vary widely. They also found that there is a potential for over-treatment in that patients may seek weight-loss drugs and weight-loss surgeries despite being medically healthy.

Despite these findings, the American Medical Association (AMA) House of Delegates voted at large to override the recommendation from the committee, a decision that was largely driven by policy. Reporters who covered the decision stated that delegates felt a lot of pressure from major stakeholders. These stakeholders wanted to shift obesity to a medical model that would require treatment and have a stronger push for insurance coverage. (If you're interested in learning more, I list several books in the resource section at the end of this book that do a deep dive into this research.)

Most of what you think you know about higher weights and health risks are from studies that provide a correlation, not a causation. **There is a critical difference between correlation and causation, especially in health research.** Health studies often find correlations, but it takes much more evidence to prove causation. Just because two things are linked doesn't mean one caused the other. Jumping to conclusions can lead to bad health advice and/or policies. A popular example to illustrate the difference between correlation and causation is to imagine if researchers notice that ice cream sales and drowning rates both go up in the summer. Does that mean that ice cream causes drowning? Of course not. They're just correlated because both happen more often when it's hot outside.

More than just poorly drawn conclusions, this weight-related public health crisis has created an environment that overlooks the serious threat of eating disorders. We've been so frightened into believing in a so-called obesity epidemic that when an individual posts untouched pictures of their larger body on social media, they are demonized for "glorifying obesity." Meanwhile we praise and "like" emaciated bodies that may have been manipulated to look that way through severe restriction, purging, and/or weight loss medications, and no one points out that they're "glorifying anorexia." In fact, no one seems to bat an eye. Instead, they ask the poster for their diet plan. Here the actual (and overlooked) health crisis is the eating disorder epidemic.

According to the National Association of Eating Disorders (NEDA), thirty million Americans will have an eating disorder in their lifetime. Thirty MILLION. Eating disorders have the highest mortality rate of any mental health disorder aside from opioid addiction, and it is estimated that someone dies *every* fifty-two minutes as a direct consequence of their eating disorder. The numbers are growing, and the ages affected are getting even younger, with studies showing children as young as five years old developing some form of disordered eating. The rate of children under twelve being admitted to a hospital for eating disorders rose 119 percent in *less than a decade.*

These statistics are alarming. And yet, I would guess that when most parents take their child to the doctor, if there are any concerns related to nutrition and weight, they are from the lens of "obesity" and prediabetic concerns versus screening for any risk factors for eating disorders. Meanwhile, eating disorders are at least twenty times more prevalent in children versus type 2 diabetes. Where are the media covered health campaigns about that?

Contrary to what we've all been made to think, eating disorders are not limited to college-aged, white females. As the statistics show, **eating disorders impact all ages, races, and genders.** Eating disorders are deadly, and their prevalence is growing. Where is the outcry and outrage about this? I think we can conclude the answer lies in misinformation and weight stigma. The good news is that the truth is spreading. When I first entered the field of eating disorders, there were probably a dozen books on the subject of diet culture. Now there is a rapidly growing community of health professionals and people in the general public who are spreading the word via books, podcasts, and social media. Clearly this information resonates, and we want more of it.

The Price We Pay

Our bodies have been judged as good or bad since the dawn of man. The judgment continues to get worse and more confusing. The ideal body went from voluptuous to heroin chic, from toned to toned-but-curvy. And how are these messages passed down? Through the media, of course. We as a society are obsessed with the weight changes of countless celebrities. I hate to contribute to the focus on the weight of public figures so I won't name names, but from my experience, most of us can name ten celebrities who've had fluctuations in their size and weight because of the media obsession over appearance.

But this kind of attention isn't just focused on celebrities; we comment on each other's appearance, most of the time with good intentions. Also, we probably all have a relative who noticed which cousin gained weight in college or who didn't lose all of the pounds brought on by pregnancy. Yet when our attention snaps to appearance, we inevitably wind up comparing ourselves to others, either consciously or subconsciously. While this comparison is undoubtedly harmful despite its normalcy, we participate anyway because we crave connection with others. We want to be part of the group. Being a member of a tribe is how we've survived throughout history. There is no shortage of research on the necessity of connection to others for both our physical and mental health.

When we consider that interconnectedness is a universal truth among most major religions and faith systems, we can begin to understand why we play along when maybe we'd rather talk or think about something other than weight and size. We can also begin to understand the potential for harm when we don't speak out against those behaviors. For example, in Islam, the oneness of God *(tawhid)* extends to creation itself and everything exists in harmony as a reflection of divine unity. Judaism teaches that all humans share the same divine spark and moral responsibility to one another. In Indigenous spiritual traditions, the idea of the "Web of Life" is a central and sacred truth that teaches that all beings are interconnected. Buddhism calls this interdependence *pratītya-samutpāda* (dependent origination), or the understanding that nothing exists in isolation, and that compassion arises naturally when we see that our well-being is bound up with all life. From a scientific perspective, an abundance of research has demonstrated that connection is a protective factor for both our physical and mental health. These include calming the body's stress systems, reducing inflammation, strengthening immunity, improving heart and brain health, supporting emotional regulation and resilience, and even increasing longevity. Both the Universe and the research agree that we need connection to one another. Comparison robs us of that.

You'll hear me say what I'm about to say more than once, but my hope is that instead of it sounding redundant, you will interpret it as reassuring: *None of this behavior or mindset is your fault.* We've all grown up in the same society where diet culture, toxic as it is, is not only common, it's at times seen as a way to connect to others. Consider how often you hear talk about dieting and weight loss. Perhaps at work, you have colleagues who are on the same newest fad diet and are constantly comparing notes. Or perhaps your company even sends out monthly communications about the weight-loss program that they unwittingly disguise as an employee health benefit. Or maybe you're out to dinner with your friends, and while you're perusing the menu, your companions start to discuss the fat or calories in the offerings or say things like, "I've had such a bad day today, I'm going to be bad tonight," or" I ate so much this past weekend, I need to be good tonight." On the other side of this kind of conversation are the seemingly complimentary comments about weight. Think about the family gatherings where everyone commented on your cousin who lost a bunch of weight, and they kept congratulating her and saying how amazing she looked.

These are just a few of the countless examples of how diet culture permeates our everyday lives in very "normal" ways. In fact, these behaviors have become so normalized that to not participate in such conversations may actually appear abnormal. Can you imagine going out to dinner with your friends and saying, "Let's just enjoy each other's company tonight and not worry about food choices." Or in the scenario of your cousin's weight loss, saying something like, "You always look beautiful, and maybe we shouldn't be commenting on each other's bodies." Feels weird? Not surprising. A possible consequence of not participating in diet culture conversations is losing connection with a group. Because of this risk, perpetuating the myth that weight matters above all else seems a small price to pay to be a part of the group.

Rather than building relationships, though, what we create with this myth perpetuation is a disconnect. We create a disconnect between our faith and souls and our bodies, its wants and needs versus an intersection that supports them all in harmony. It's a disconnect from being present in the moment due to ruminations in the mind, a disconnect from meaningful conversations that lead to deeper connections, and a disconnect from what God wants for us in this one short life we have been blessed with on Earth, and that is our one true purpose.

Diet Culture Negatively Affects All Aspects of Living

Right about now, you may be thinking, *Whoa, okay, this all sounds very familiar, and if I'm honest with myself, I agree with a lot of this. But isn't it true that losing weight is healthier than not trying to lose weight?*

Well, let's dissect that. First, we have to come to an agreement about what the definition of "health" is before we can proceed. The WHO constitution states that "Health is a state of complete physical, mental, and social well-being and not merely the absence of disease or infirmity." I actually think this is a fair definition. You'll notice that it doesn't solely call out the status of one's physical health but also includes both mental and social well-being. So let's start with mental health.

How Our Mental and Social Health Suffers

I think we can all agree that endless dieting, ruminating about calories or macros, and obsessing about the numbers on your scale and the size tag of your pants does not lead to optimal mental health. The only argument I've ever heard against this is that people have more confidence when they are at a smaller weight. To which I say, of course you do. Our society celebrates weight loss. However, as we've learned and will discuss in more depth, weight loss is temporary 95 percent of the time. Therefore, relying on the confidence of weight loss to boost your mental health is shaky ground to stand on.

There is a lot of research about how dieting affects mental health, the most recent findings reported in the journal *BMJ Nutrition, Prevention & Health*. It tells us that dieting can at the very least lead to frustration, stress, and low self-esteem. At worst, dieting can lead to clinically diagnosed depression and anxiety. Why? The vast majority of folks who attempt to intentionally lose weight will not be able to keep it off. An estimated 5 percent will be able to sustain intentional weight loss. So if you're not in that 5 percent, then you are forever climbing an uphill battle in which you will never reach the summit. And heartbreakingly, you'll blame yourself for it because the marketing dollars behind these weight-loss products will make sure you don't blame them.

Now for our social well-being. Here's a game of Have You Ever. Have you ever:

- Skipped out on a social event because you didn't think there would be any "safe" foods to eat?
- Skipped out on a social event because you didn't think you had anything to wear that you felt good in (read "look thin in")?
- Found yourself distracted from conversation because of worries about appearance or what food was being served?
- Avoided the beach, lake, or pool because of the fear of being seen in a bathing suit?
- Delayed dating or sexual intimacy because you didn't feel attractive because you were "heavier" than you wanted to be?

- Brought a dish to a party or BBQ that was deliberately aligned with your current diet? (I'm reminded of the episode of Friends where Brad Pitt joins the gang for Thanksgiving and brings the no-fat, no-sugar, no-dairy dessert because he's trying to maintain his weight loss. If you recall, he tells them to throw it out because it's no good.)

And have you ever found that any of these avoidance behaviors brought you joy, deepened your relationships, or made you feel good in any way, shape, or form?

Not only does diet culture hurt our social relationships, it also holds us back from love and intimacy. I've had many patients over the years describe substantial insecurities as a result of not having the "ideal" body, from putting themselves out there to start dating all the way to being intimate with their partner. Many individuals delay dating until they achieve their desired weight, resulting in prolonged isolation and loneliness. Others insist on turning the lights off before undressing despite body reassurance from partners, feeling self-conscious even with the person they trust the most in the world.

I hope you see where I'm going. There are endless ways in which diet culture impacts our social well-being in a negative way. And according to the WHO, that's not health.

Again, No, the Number on the Scale Does Not Measure Actual Health

Remember Anne and Veronica? You cannot look at a person and determine their health based on their weight. The most accepted method for determining health is an overall combination of health metrics including blood pressure, blood sugar, cholesterol, heart rate, hormone levels, and so on. These metrics can be improved via positive behavior habits, such as sleep, exercise, and nutrition, even when no weight is lost. If weight is lost as a result of those behaviors, the weight loss becomes the hero of the improved metrics, not the behaviors themselves.

At this point, you might ask, *Is there research that determines that weight loss can have a positive impact on (fill in the blank) condition?* Absolutely. But was it the sheer outcome of being a lower number on the scale that led to improved metrics? Or was it the targeted lifestyle behavior? If someone gets a severe stomach virus and loses 5 percent of their body weight in a week because they can't keep food down, would we assume their health markers improved? Of course not. The sheer lower number on the scale would not indicate an improvement in biomarkers. Therefore, we must get to the place where we accept that it is the behaviors that impact our health, completely and totally, regardless of our weight.

Additionally, the physical consequences of weight cycling have been well researched. Weight cycling is when a person repeatedly loses weight and then gains it back, often through dieting. It's also sometimes called *yo-yo dieting* as the weight goes up and down like a yo-yo. For so many of us, this is repeated so often throughout our lives and the lives of people we know that it seems normal. But just because something is common doesn't necessarily mean it's healthy for our bodies.

Weight cycling can lead to metabolic disturbances, including changes in insulin sensitivity and glucose metabolism. Repeated weight loss and regain may negatively affect the beta cells in the pancreas, which produce insulin, which could raise the risk of developing type 2 diabetes. Weight cycling has also been linked to increased cardiovascular risks, including hypertension, heart disease, and stroke. The most recent study, published in December 2025, comes from the *Journal of Clinical Endocrinology & Metabolism.* This study reviewed the health records of over 83,000 adults. Compared with adults whose weight remained stable, adults whose weight had cycled had significantly higher risks of several conditions, including heart failure, obstructive sleep apnea, metabolic dysfunction–associated steatotic liver disease, and type 2 diabetes. These findings call into question weight-focused health models by showing that repeated weight loss and regain may independently increase health risks, highlighting the need for sustainable, non-diet approaches. If you're noticing that those same conditions are supposed to be resolved with weight loss, then your confusion is understandable.

If you are interested, there are multiple sources that dive into specific conditions and the oversimplifications that weight loss resulted in improvement in said condition. For the purposes of this book, suffice to say that you have been misled (through no fault of your own) to believe that weight loss is the singular path to health. I also hope you can hear that the evidence does not support black and white statements, and that there are very real, evidence-based consequences emotionally, socially, and yes, physically. And again, that's not health.

The Role of Social Determinants

Beyond mental and social health, the WHO also recognizes what's known as Social Determinants of Health, or SDOH for short. SDOH are the conditions in which people are born, grow, live, work, and age and how they affect their overall health and quality of life. These include economic stability, education access and quality, health care access and quality, neighborhood and environment, and social and community context. Some studies suggest SDOH accounts for 30 percent and up to as much as 90 percent of health outcomes. Yet rarely are these aspects evaluated and accounted for in healthcare. We'll address this again in later chapters.

Real, Hard-Earned Money Costs

Finally, if we look at the literal cost of health, consider for a moment the amount of money you have spent on gym memberships, weight-loss food products, shakes, supplements, drugs, surgery, and so on. While we can't go back in time and get that money back for you, **you can decide today, right now at this moment, that you will never give another one of your hard-earned dollars to a company that makes millions off of telling you that you're not good enough exactly as you are.**

While you're at it, direct a few of those dollars towards a couple of items of clothing that make you feel good, that are your style, and, most importantly, that are comfortable. Friends, I realize we're just getting started together, but I hope you know by now that you deserve better than jeans that are so tight they dig into your waist every time you sit or an underwire bra that leaves a deep mark after you've removed it at the end of the day. *You shouldn't feel guilty for buying clothing that fits.* Period.

And if you're short on cash, explore the fun and exciting world of thrifting. One of my favorite sweaters and one of my favorite dresses were thrifted. They are classic and comfortable and I get compliments on them all the time. The point is, don't waste another day in discomfort or pain. Buy the bigger size. Give yourself some much deserved peace. And let's all enter our comfort era together.

The Dangers of Fat Phobia

Before we move on to the next principle, we need to spend some time looking at how diet culture has created the concept of fat phobia and how that has resulted in discrimination and oppression of people in larger bodies.

When it comes to talking about size, there are many amazing activists who currently use the word *fat* in an effort to neutralize the word and eliminate any negative connotation in the same way that *short, tall, blond hair, freckles,* and so on are all neutral descriptors. However, as this word is still triggering for some, and this writer currently occupies what's known as a straight-sized body type, it feels appropriate to use "smaller" and "larger" bodies as descriptors. Now why would someone who does not live in a larger body type care about this? Firstly, I care about all people and have always been sensitive to, and to the best of my ability, I'm an ally for marginalized groups. I've been a social worker for over twenty years. That, combined with my faith, demands that I stand up for the oppressed. Make no mistake, people who live in larger bodies are an oppressed group.

People in larger bodies report significant discrimination beginning as young as early childhood that continues throughout their lives. A 2011 study published in the *Journal of Adolescent Health* reports that fat-shaming is the number one type of bullying in school-age children. This same study surveyed over 1,500 high school students and found that approximately 41 percent identified being "overweight" as the primary reason for bullying, surpassing other factors such as sexual orientation, intelligence, race, and physical disability. Another study in 2010 from the *American Journal of Public Health* reports that discrimination against people of larger body types is equal to the stress of discrimination against other marginalized groups.

Suffice to say, we are a fat-phobic society. Some believe that people in larger bodies are lazy and don't have enough willpower to "do the work" of dieting and exercise. As such, it is socially acceptable to shame people on airplanes or in the grocery store or at the gym or really anywhere through the guise of offering helpful "advice." Ask any larger person about the health trolls, and they'll have endless stories for you.

Health trolls are people who subscribe to "healthism," which is the belief that morality is tied to health. They feel superior to others for what they believe are misguided health choices. If you get nothing else from this book, don't be a health troll. Other people's health and bodies are none of our business. This isn't Sandi's command; this is God's command. I can't say I've ever seen the phrase "health troll" in any sacred text; however, across all religions, we are called to care for one another and to show compassion and love to our neighbors. In Hinduism, all beings are manifestations of *Brahman,* the universal soul, reminding us that to harm another is to harm ourselves. This will mean unlearning some misinformation and pausing before spreading that misinformation, no matter how well-intended. We can each do a better job of leading with kindness. Martin Luther King Jr. said it best: "The ultimate tragedy is not the oppression and cruelty by the bad people but the silence over that by the good people."

In today's society, there are many reasons why living in a thinner body can be seen as an advantage. So, who can blame anyone for wanting to be thinner? The reality is that thinner people are often treated better. They're more likely to be hired and to hold higher-paying jobs. They receive more compliments, and people make positive assumptions about them, such as being disciplined, active, and self-controlled. They tend to receive better healthcare, experience greater social acceptance, and avoid the harsh reality of anti-fat bias.

At one point in my thirties, I went through a terrible period of depression. It lasted several months, and I could not get out from under it. I was sad every day and was frequently tearful. I felt helpless and worthless, as if a black cloud followed me around wherever I went. I was able to eventually pull myself out with the help of medication, therapy, and the love of the handful of friends and family I opened up to. But a side effect that no one questioned was my rapid weight loss.

I had zero appetite. Zero, even though I've loved and appreciated food my entire life. I forced myself to eat enough only to avoid terrible headaches. Food tasted like cardboard, and my stomach was always nauseous. I shrank very noticeably. Yet no one, not a single person, ever asked me if anything was wrong. On the contrary, I was bombarded with compliments and attention. I wish I had the language I do now to have been honest with everyone. I wish I could've said, "I know you think you're being kind, but I'm not okay. I'm shrinking because I can barely get out of bed in the morning. That's not a thing to praise." I share this story to say that compliments about weight loss are dangerous. Not only does it perpetuate the idea that thinner is better, but **we can never have any idea what is going on for folks behind closed doors or what is going on medically or emotionally that may have caused the weight loss.** They may be in the grips of crisis, but instead of focusing on the heart and mind of the person, we're congratulating them on getting "beach body ready."

In short, thin privilege is real, and it operates on both a subconscious and societal level. It makes logical sense that people in larger bodies would desire to be in smaller ones. Yet, like any oppressed group, it should never be on those individuals to conform to society's version of an ideal norm. It's society's attitude towards people in larger bodies and anti-fat bias that needs to change.

If that seems like a daunting undertaking, you are correct. How do we get society to change its point of view? Part of it is understanding the broader context of diet culture, and the other part is how it connects to a patriarchal society. Women's bodies have been objectified, scrutinized, and policed throughout history as patriarchal systems seek to control and regulate female autonomy. Diet culture perpetuates the idea that women must conform to narrow beauty standards in order to be valued and accepted.

In a patriarchal society, women are often valued primarily for their physical appearance, particularly their adherence to ideals of thinness, youth, and beauty. This leads to the belief that women's worth is determined by their body size and shape, fueling the pressure to conform to these standards through restrictive diets and exercise regimens. Diet culture thrives in a patriarchal society not only because of societal expectations of women's bodies, but also from profiting off women's insecurities around meeting those expectations. Industries like diet, beauty, and fitness capitalize on the idea that women's bodies need to be "fixed," selling products and services that promise to help women shrink their bodies to meet societal expectations. This creates a cycle where women are encouraged to continuously consume weight-loss products in pursuit of the ideal (and ever-changing) standard of beauty that is never truly attainable.

As you can imagine, the impact of diet culture isn't felt equally by all women. Women of color, LGBTQ+ individuals, and those from lower-income backgrounds often face additional challenges. For women of color, diet culture is often compounded by racialized beauty standards that favor Eurocentric features and body types. As a result, women of color are often excluded from mainstream beauty ideals, which can lead to feelings of inadequacy and an increased desire to conform to a standard that does not reflect their natural bodies. Author Sabrina Strings takes this to a much deeper level in her book, *Fearing the Black Body: The Racial Origins of Fat Phobia.* This must-read provides an eye-opening historical account that the thin ideal is not neutral or even purely health-based, but rather, it's rooted in anti-Blackness. She provides extensive research that demonstrates how fat phobia was built through racial and moral hierarchies that continue to shape diet culture today.

Further, LGBTQ+ individuals face their own set of challenges in diet culture, often driven by societal expectations related to gender norms and roles. For trans and non-binary individuals, the pressure to conform to traditional gendered ideals of beauty can be particularly intense. The desire to match a gender identity that feels authentic while also meeting societal expectations of how one should look often creates deep internal conflict. For example, trans women may face pressure to maintain a slim, traditionally feminine body, while trans men may feel the pressure to adopt a more muscular, masculine appearance, which may not align with their authentic body experiences or the realities of hormone therapy.

Finally, lower-income individuals face barriers that are often overlooked in discussions about diet culture. Financial constraints make it difficult to access the resources necessary to maintain a diet that aligns with society's expectations of health and beauty. Organic foods, gym memberships, and personal trainers are often out of reach for those in economically disadvantaged communities. Moreover, food insecurity and limited access to healthy, affordable options in low-income neighborhoods can force people to rely on processed, cheap foods, which are often stigmatized as "unhealthy" within diet culture. This can perpetuate a cycle of body dissatisfaction, as they are unable to meet the standards of health and beauty that diet culture promotes, which further entrenches the idea that their worth is linked to their appearance.

These compounded challenges highlight the need to recognize diverse experiences, especially when addressing the harmful effects of diet culture. Women of color, LGBTQ+ individuals, and lower-income women all face unique barriers that go beyond personal choice or behavior; these are deeply rooted in systemic inequality, social exclusion, and the perpetuation of unrealistic beauty standards. By acknowledging these intersecting identities, we can create a more inclusive dialogue around body image and work to dismantle the harmful impact of diet culture for all people, regardless of race, gender, or socioeconomic status.

It's worth noting that those with the most power benefit greatly by keeping us distracted. If we're worried about our bodies, we won't have time to worry about our rights. Our attention is a powerful resource. Entire industries exist because we are taught to focus on our perceived flaws and constant self-improvement. When so much energy is directed toward self-surveillance, there is very little left for courage, creativity, advocacy, or community. **What if instead of focusing on changing our bodies, we put one hundred percent of our energy into changing the world?** Can. You. Imagine.

We've spent a long time on the first principle of intuitive eating, and for good reason: While the other principles don't necessarily have to be addressed or worked on in chronological order (other than the first one and last one), we really can't have much success without first working on rejecting diet culture. You have to come to some place of acceptance around the truths and lies about diet culture. This will not be a perfect journey. There will be times when you will feel really angry about diet culture. Nearly all of us who go through this process go through a phase where we are frankly pissed off at the lies we were told and the heart-breaking amount of wasted time, effort, shame, and guilt. Give yourself grace as you cope with this new information and your own self-reflection. As the author, Nobel laureate, and Holocaust survivor Elie Wiesel wrote, "Every question [possesses] a power that [does not] lie in the answer." Questions challenge assumptions and provoke critical thinking. Even if we never find definitive answers, the journey of self-reflection alone can lead to deeper insights and clarity in direction.

You have likely been on the diet culture train for decades, so don't be surprised when you start to second guess yourself or feel resistant to change. Buddhism teaches that "no one saves us but ourselves. No one can and no one may. We ourselves must walk the path." (*The Dhammapada,* Verse 165.) You can go as slow as feels right for you. Just don't give up. The hard and scary place of doing and thinking something new is exactly where transformation is born. "Do not despise these small beginnings, for the Lord rejoices to see the work begin." (Zechariah 4:10 NLT)

You've already taken a huge first step by picking up this book and reading this far. There is a part of you that is ready for change even if it's partnered with feelings of doubt or confusion. But I'd also love to provide you with this reassurance: There is reason to allow yourself feelings of hope. **Every food rule you release and every diet-culture advertisement, comment, and negative inner thought that you challenge is a step toward freedom.** This work allows you to reconnect with your faith in a deeply personal way and to begin seeing your body not as a problem to fix, but as a sacred gift to care for just as it is today.

As you let go of the external pressures of diet culture and embrace your inherent worth, you open space for peace, connection, and deeper spirituality. On the other side of diet culture is an opportunity to live in alignment with the divine and to step into a life that truly honors both your physical and spiritual being. There are so many reasons to have hope, so give yourself permission to allow hope to flourish. The absence of diet culture will make way for an abundance of gratitude, presence, and connection, allowing your faith to guide you toward a life of wholeness, joy, and spiritual harmony. Once you've cleared out the noise of diet culture, the Universe is ready to rush in.

Practice Rejecting Diet Culture

It's not easy to reject what might be a lifetime of diet culture, but it's crucial if you want to live a better life, the one that's always been meant for you. So the first step? Awareness. Make note of every time you hear or see something related to diet culture. This includes commercials, online advertisements, social media influencers, comments on television, conversations in the real world. You will be astounded at the frequency once you start looking.

Notice how often diet talk comes up in your life, whether in conversation or in your thoughts, and then consciously choose not to engage with it. Just as in some mediation practices, we're not aiming to control our thoughts or others' conversations. All you need to do is simply notice when diet talk comes up and allow it to pass on through without judgment or comment. It will be difficult at first because it's a natural response to want to join in. But the next time a coworker or friend or family member starts commenting about their weight, someone else's weight, the latest diet they're trying, or anything remotely related to diet culture, let the conversation go. If it's just the two of you, try steering the chat in another direction. If you're in a group, stay silent or walk away. It's up to you. But do your best not to engage. Use your breath to talk about something much more meaningful to you than perpetuating negative self-talk.

Second step? Cleanse your mind and physical space. Get rid of your dieting books, cancel your subscriptions to diet magazines, throw out the diet food, donate the "aspirational" clothes, and toss the scale (or at least hide it somewhere you can't easily access it if you're not ready to toss it). Also, unfollow any influencer on social media who is pushing the diet culture narrative and replace them with creators who promote intuition, embodiment, compassion, or spiritual grounding. We want to let go of the things that are telling us we're not good enough just as we are.

Take time to experiment with this process as well. Maybe you choose to eliminate one thing a day versus all at once. Or, if you're ready to do a one-and-done purge, then go for it and do a complete overhaul.

As you go through this cleansing process, one thing to consider is starting a journal. It's natural to have a lot of emotions and memories (good and bad) surface during this process, and writing helps you sort it out. For this reason, I include reflection questions and action items at the end of each chapter. For this chapter, take time to write about how it feels to know that there's nothing wrong with or bad about your size and shape.

- How does it feel to reject diet culture and all of its trappings?
- Do you feel a bit lost without counting calories?
- Have you started to remember what it feels like to ask yourself, "What do I want to eat?" instead of following a chart that tells you what you should eat?
- In what ways has diet culture shaped how you measure your own worth, and how does that differ from how your faith or spiritual beliefs define your worth?

- What moments from your past dieting experiences stand out as emotionally painful or exhausting, and what do those memories reveal about what you truly want for your life moving forward?
- When you imagine accepting your biology and releasing the pursuit of intentional weight loss, what emotions arise?
- When you reflect on New Year's resolutions, how many times have they included a change in your weight? How long did they last?
- What was your most recent resolution, and what would be different if weight loss weren't the goal?

If journaling isn't your thing, maybe bring up these questions with a friend or loved one, your therapist or spiritual advisor. Or maybe you simply ponder these in an intentional period of silence and meditation.

After you've reflected, discussed, or written about what's coming up for you, don't forget to spend time on what excites you about this process. You're taking your life back, inside and out. What will you do with all of your free time? What will you get to read now that your library queue isn't full of diet books? What new activity do you want to try that you've held back from because of the misperceptions you have about your current weight? What recipe have you read over and over but haven't cooked because of the amount of butter in it? Guess what? Now's the time to pull it out and give it a try. Your future suddenly looks like a Costco sample day: abundant, surprising, and weirdly delightful.

Chapter Three

Honor Your Hunger and Trust the Design

Have you ever been "hangry"? If you know, you know. I once stood at an intersection of a street in Colmar, France, completely paralyzed with indecision about which way to go and unreasonably frustrated despite being in one of the most beautiful cities in the world. My muscles were tight, and I was inexplicably irritable, seemingly out of nowhere. Every question asked of me resulted in a brusque, "I don't know!" I could hear the snippiness in my voice.

My husband wisely made the decision for us to stop in at a nearby restaurant opening for the day. After tearing through the *assiette de fromages* recommended by our server, there is a humorous photo of me taken less than fifteen minutes later where I look so happy. (The *assiette de fromages* was the perfect cheese plate of both soft and hard cheeses served with dried fruits, assorted nuts, and, of course, a freshly sliced, crisp baguette. It was heaven on a plate.) You would never have guessed that I'd been cranky. Everything was right with the world again.

What had changed? What could explain a total transformation in mood and behavior? You guessed it. I had been *hangry*—irritable and angry because of hunger. This affliction comes on suddenly. You didn't even realize you were hungry, but then all of a sudden, you become irrationally agitated and snap at anyone who has the great misfortune of crossing your path. In mere seconds, the people you love most in the world have become the most annoying humans on the planet. Heaven forbid it occurs while you're driving, and someone cuts you off. I'm convinced it is at the root of most road rage incidents, which is why I've repurposed the center console of my car into a non-perishable snack compartment. (It's a brilliant idea, and you're welcome to steal it. It saves lives.)

It's also why for the last several years of our marriage, before my husband walks into the convenience store at the gas station for coffee, he asks me if I want anything. I say, "No," and he asks, "Are you sure?" I say, "Yes, I'm sure," and he still comes out with a snack for me. There are times when I legitimately do not want the snack because we've just eaten, are about to eat, or I'm simply not hungry. But other times, I don't realize I need a snack until he's back in the car holding it out to me. Because of this, he's grown to see the snack as a life preserver—you pray you never need it, but you'll be very glad you have it if you do.

Why does this happen? How is it possible to be a completely loving, affectionate, and rational human being one minute and then the human equivalent of a Venus flytrap the next? Three reasons: First, because diet culture has taught us to ignore signs of hunger; second, we do not adequately acknowledge our hunger signs; and third, we don't even know what hunger signs are. We start getting nutrition information in school as early as preschool—"A is for Apple, and apples are good for you"—but as we get older, we aren't taught about the phases of hunger signs.

You know the saying that if you feel thirsty, you are likely already a glass of water behind? The same is true for food. The truth is that by the time we start *feeling* our stomachs grumble, we've already gone too long without food. The diet culture "rules" of food have conditioned us not to listen to our body's signals. And frankly, we don't want to listen because the less we eat the better, right? Wrong.

The next principle of intuitive eating that we'll discuss is "honor your hunger," which sounds like it should be the easiest principle of all. We all feel hungry, so we should eat when we feel that hunger. Done. Next chapter. If only it were so simple. Diet culture has conditioned us to disrespect our hunger, or perhaps more specifically, to distrust it. Taking it further, when we mistrust what our body is telling us, we're not just dismissing or ignoring the need for fuel; we're actively mistrusting God's intelligent design for our vessel. **Our bodies are not just happy accidents; they were created with complex mechanisms that all work in harmony,** as long as we do our part in keeping them in good working order through actions like eating and drinking.

Think of it like this: When we feel hungry, we tend to first ask ourselves a bunch of questions:

- *Am I really hungry, or am I just thirsty?*
- *Has it been long enough since I last ate and therefore reasonable for me to be hungry again?*
- *Am I just feeling bored? Frustrated? Depressed?*
- *Is there anything "safe" for me to eat right now if I decide to eat?*
- *What have I eaten already today? How many calories have I already had? Have I saved enough calories throughout the day so that I'm allowed to eat again now?*
- *What were my macros at the last meal?*

Wow. It's just exhausting! And let's remember that this is a biological need for survival that we are questioning. Imagine you realize that you suddenly need to relieve your bladder. This sensation arrives multiple times a day, as it has every day since birth. But now you ask yourself: *Do I really have to pee? I've already peed twice today, so surely I don't have to pee again? The last time I peed was only a few hours ago. I shouldn't pee again, it's too soon.* We could take this analogy further, but you get the point. Instead of questioning our bodies' biological need for food, we need to learn to honor its inherent wisdom and the intelligent, complex design that wants us to survive and thrive. After all, **it's impossible to live out our purpose if we're too weak or distracted from ignoring our hunger.**

Food and Function

Our bodies are amazing, and we'll discuss all of those amazing ways in Chapter 9, "Respect Your Body and Have Reverence for Your Sacred Vessel," but for now, I want to point out how resourceful they are when it comes to survival. If you don't eat today, tomorrow, or the day after that, you can survive. And if you have access to water, you can likely survive for several weeks. But what's actually happening inside the body when it's hungry?

Our bodies usually use glucose, or sugar, as the main source of energy. After one day without food, those reserves are likely depleted, so on day two or three, the body will begin breaking down fatty acids for fuel. But once those fatty acid reserves are gone, usually within one week without food, the body will start breaking down muscle to obtain protein. As the breakdown of muscle continues into the second week of not eating, we begin to lose heart, kidney and liver function. Again, assuming you have water, this can last for another few weeks, but for most of us, even with water, we would die from malnutrition and its complications in less than two months.

The truth is that most diets do not allow you (or tell you) to eat enough. Period. They're interested in restricting as much as possible for short-term weight loss "rewards" so that you keep giving them money. In fact, some mainstream diets have their customers eating only 1,200 calories per day. To put this in perspective, according to the American Dietetics Association, 1,200 calories is the recommended daily allowance for a toddler (or a large dog). That is an insufficient number of calories for a grown human. Considering the human body needs at least 1,400 calories a day simply to sustain its Basal Metabolic Rate (BMR), an adult eating only enough to sustain a toddler is *not enough*. While BMR is highly individualized, a general range is between 1,200-1,800 for the body to perform life-sustaining functions when completely at rest, things like breathing, blood circulation, blood temperature regulation, digestion, and brain function. You know, processes that keep you alive. Eating below BMR tells your body you are in starvation mode.

Starvation has been used as a method of torture throughout history to control, punish, and psychologically break prisoners. It's one of the oldest weapons of war. By deliberately depriving individuals of food, captors weaken the body, cloud judgment, and increase vulnerability. We've seen it employed in prisons, wartime camps, and political oppression to break resistance, force compliance, or inflict suffering. In fact, starvation of a civilian population is considered a war crime, a crime against humanity, or an act of genocide according to modern international criminal law. So the diet that cuts your calories below your individual BMR is an act of war against self. Think about that.

The Ongoing Study of Starvation

Sandi, you might be thinking, *I get it. Starving the body is terrible. But I'm not starving myself; I'm just cutting back on a few calories to slim down for (insert holiday or event here). It's really not a big deal.*

Except that the human body can't tell the difference between starvation and dieting. I know it can seem innocuous to skip a meal or a snack here and there, but to the body, it can be devastating.

Nutrition and the study of food and the body became topics of interest for governments all over the world during World Wars I and II. It was crucial to have a healthy population in order to have a strong military presence and home front supporting those military efforts. As the world came out of these devastating wars, we were still interested in how treatments like starvation affected the body and how to help a starved body effectively recover. And so scientists and researchers at the University of Minnesota developed the now infamous Minnesota Starvation Study, conducted from November 1944 to December 1945.

This study has been cited in many publications because of its profound implications, but here are the highlights. Two hundred men from the Civilian Public Service volunteered for a starvation study to research famine as part of the war effort. Researchers selected thirty-six healthy subjects who took part in the study that included a 24-week starvation period. Critical to note, at this time, starvation meant reducing the men's daily caloric intake to under 1600 calories. (As we've already discussed but is worth repeating, several mainstream diets recommend restrictions way below this number.)

So did the men eventually get used to feeling hungry and rejoice in their slimmer bodies and reduced pant sizes? You might be wondering. No, that was definitely not the case.

Some of the men were unable to complete the study because the restrictions felt too severe. The remaining subjects experienced traumatic outcomes, which was not altogether surprising. They reported extreme discomfort, preoccupation and obsession with food, confusion, disorientation, reduced sex drive, social withdrawal and isolation, and depression, with one severe example of self-mutilation.

If you have ever been on a restrictive diet, it is highly likely you have experienced many of those symptoms as well. And what's heartbreaking is that we choose to do this to ourselves. Willingly. Intentionally. Because we've been misled about what health really means.

Fast forward to late 1968 when a weight loss camp for children opened their flagship location in Ferndale, New York. Camp Shane grew to fame and notoriety due to the plague of diet culture and fat phobia with endorsements from celebrities and the media. Kids were only spending six weeks of their summer at the camp and losing a ton of weight.

Unfortunately, no one seemed to be concerned about *how* they were losing so much weight. And this went on for decades. Growing kids and teenagers would work out and stay active for eight to ten hours a day, and be restricted to less than 1,000 calories a day. The kids became obsessed with food. They would find ways to sneak it in. Food became the currency at camp and mini black markets sprang up. Food was used for bribes, and in some of the camp's darkest days, used in exchanges for sexual encounters since the kids were often unsupervised. The camp finally closed its doors in 2021, and many of the campers who survived the experience admit to a lifelong struggle with their bodies and their relationships with food. If it breaks your heart that children were subjected to this torture for fifty years, it should. But weight loss camps and "fat camps" still exist. This is the legacy of diet culture.

Finding a Way Back to Myself

When I was in college, I heard about the "freshman fifteen," but as a historically slim young woman—and I know this in and of itself gives me a fair amount of privilege—I wasn't very concerned. I consider myself fortunate that dieting hadn't permeated my existence yet. After college, though, I moved to Florida for a job and suddenly began to see a number of changes in my body shape and size, including a few extra pounds. When I returned home to New

Jersey, the changes I noticed but weren't wildly concerned about became much more concerning when everyone else pointed them out to me.

Next thing I know, I'm attending Weight Watchers (rebranded as WW) meetings every Wednesday evening with my family. That complete change in framework for me about eating (or not eating) for weight loss created shame and guilt around food and body shape and size. Thinking about my body and food so differently sadly turned into almost ten years of disordered eating. Dieting actually remains the number one predictor for developing a future eating disorder. In 1999, the *British Medical Journal* published the findings of a three-year study that followed 2,500 teenage girls and found that girls who reported severe dieting were eighteen times more likely to develop eating disorders than those who did not diet. **Even moderate dieting was associated with a fivefold increase in the incidence of eating disorders.**

A word about self-disclosure. As a therapist, we're trained that self-disclosure (sharing personal details about oneself to a patient) should only be done sparingly and when it has an intentional positive purpose for that patient. That said, it's still subjective, and there is a spectrum in terms of the use and frequency of self-disclosure. I'm a one on a scale of one to ten, with ten being frequent use of self-disclosure. In fact, I can remember very clearly the two times I have chosen to share anything personal about myself with a patient. While I realize that you, reader, are not one of my patients, it's still a very big leap for me to tell my personal stories. But a good friend told me that I need to share why this work is important to me. I have a personal investment in my desire to dismantle diet culture outside of my purpose-driven work as a clinician.

So here we go.

Those ten years were marked with many different highlights and lowlights, just as all of us have within a decade of life. I was single. I was married. I got divorced. I had multiple different jobs and made a lot of friends at those jobs. But throughout all of it, every day, I got on a scale in the morning and let that scale tell me not only how I was doing as a person, but what kind of a day I would have. The number on the scale totally and completely defined my sense of self and self-worth. Here I am many years later in a very healthy place with food and my body, and I can still look at a picture during that time period and remember how much I weighed because it was such a part of my identity. If you're making the assumption that I was not honoring my hunger during those years, you would be completely correct.

While I never met the criteria for an eating disorder, I absolutely exhibited disordered eating behaviors. What's the difference, you may ask? According to the Diagnostic and Statistical Manual of Mental Disorders (DSM), aka the handbook for mental health clinicians, there are a handful of conditions that consist of multiple criteria that, when met, are defined as an eating disorder, such as anorexia nervosa, bulimia, and binge eating disorder. Only a mental health professional, preferably one who has eating disorder expertise or credentials like a Certified Eating Disorder Specialist (CEDS), can make the official diagnosis. But suffice it to say, at the time, I was still struggling.

I kept myself on a very strict low-calorie diet for years and obsessed about food and my body shape and size. In fact, I held my hunger as a badge of honor. As shameful as it is to admit now , if I was hungry, that meant I had willpower. Sad, I know.

I can remember seeing a dietician at one point. I wish I could say it was because I knew I wasn't getting enough nutrition, but the truth is, I was weight cycling and wanted the weight to stay off. When she told me (justifiably) that I wasn't eating enough throughout the day and wanted me to eat more, I never saw her again.

There were days I was devastated about my body and my weight and saw myself as a complete failure because I wasn't the version of thin I thought I should be, no matter what size I was at any given time. I got sucked into the idea that thinner was better and held a preoccupation that was very psychologically damaging.

As I sit here today in a coffee shop with my decaf coffee and chocolate chip cookie, I can say that I don't even recognize that girl anymore. **My life has been transformed by making peace with food and my body.** And while everyone's path is different, my personal journey can be credited to the principles of intuitive eating and a gut belief that God did not want me to live like that.

The Multiple Sides of Fasting

There's a story in the Bible about Jesus feeding five thousand. The story goes that a large crowd shows up to hear Jesus teach. His disciples are like, "Yo, Jesus, these people are hungry," and Jesus tells them to feed the people. A young boy gives Jesus five loaves of bread and two fish, and the miracle is that after Jesus blessed the food, it fed all five thousand people, even leaving enough leftovers for twelve additional baskets.

Whether you believe in miracles or not, the symbolism is clear. Hunger is seen, valued, and heard. Jesus didn't ignore the crowd's physical hunger or scold them for being needy. He acknowledged it, took it seriously, and responded with compassion. This mirrors the principle of honoring your own hunger: listening, responding with care, and not shaming yourself for needing nourishment.

Your hunger is not an inconvenience. It's a signal from your body and is a sacred part of your design. Jesus didn't offer only spiritual teaching. He fed real bodies with real food. He recognized that spiritual and physical needs are connected. Just as Jesus responded to the crowd's hunger with compassion and abundance, we, too, can meet our own hunger with kindness, not judgment.

You may be wondering about intentional fasting for religious purposes. Let's explore that for a moment. Fasting is believed to be a practice of self-discipline, sacrifice, and self-control. It can be considered a time for preparing to commune with God and a time for deeper, sacred reflection. Many religions have this practice for a variety of reasons.

Within many Christian denominations, it is believed that adults should abstain from all meat products on Fridays during the Lenten season, and if in good health, limit overall intake on both Ash Wednesday and Good Friday. Yet even this practice has changed with the times. Historically, people were required to fast completely on those two days, but the custom has evolved to allow for one regular sized meal and two small meals, although many Catholics still follow the older traditions of fasting. Within Judaism, Yom Kippur, which is considered the most important day of the Jewish year, requires fasting for all adults who are healthy enough to participate as a means of repentance. Fasting is also common within the Hindu traditions, and followers will fast on certain days as devotees of a particular deity.

The fasting traditions within Islam are a well-known example. Fasting is obligatory for every Muslim for one entire month of the year during Ramadan. Each day, the fast begins at dawn and ends at sunset. During this time, Muslims are asked to remember those who are less fortunate than themselves. It is meant to cleanse the soul as well as bring them closer to God.

You might also ask that if there are fasting practices in many of the religions of the world, then isn't there value in fasting on a spiritual level? Well, let's note some important points. In all of the above examples, fasting is not required for children or adults who are ill or frail. This tells us that while the practice of fasting is important to honor their traditions, it is not to be practiced at the cost of one's health. Secondly, these practices are brief and meant to be conducted in the short-term. Thirdly, and most importantly, they have absolutely nothing to do with promoting intentional weight loss.

In Buddhism, there is a powerful story of the Buddha accepting rice pudding. Before his enlightenment, Siddhartha Gautama (the Buddha) was convinced that practicing extreme fasting and self-denial would lead to spiritual awakening. He became so weak he nearly died. One day, a young woman offered him a simple bowl of rice pudding. After he accepted and ate the food, he felt his strength return and realized that denying his body was not the path to wisdom. This moment marked the birth of the Middle Way, which is the understanding that true spiritual practice lies between deprivation and indulgence. It teaches that **spiritual growth requires compassion for the body as well as the mind, and that honoring hunger is not weakness but wisdom.**

Far from the purpose of religious fasting, there has been a lot of noise over the last few years about a fad diet called *intermittent fasting*, or *IF.* And yes, it is a fad diet. The term first surfaced in 2012 when a journalist wrote about his personal experience and his perceived benefits of the practice. As you can imagine, in our diet-obsessed culture, this idea quickly gained popularity without any actual scientific backing supporting his unqualified observational findings. The journalist's observational findings were his own personal impressions, not scientifically validated data. He reported that eating normally five days a week and then limiting his intake for two designated days seemed to help him lose weight, feel more focused, and experience what he believed were improvements in his overall health. These anecdotal observations were later generalized in media coverage, which contributed to the diet's explosion in popularity despite the lack of rigorous research at that point. Subsequently, by 2020, almost a quarter of Americans (approximately 62 million people) had tried this particular diet. This is a staggering figure, but when we consider our obsession with diet culture, maybe we shouldn't be so surprised.

Intermittent fasting can be confusing because there are so many methods out there. Put simply, a general definition would describe it as cycling between scheduled periods of eating and periods of not eating. Common examples include the original 5:2 pattern described above where a person eats normally for five days each week and severely limits calorie intake for two days. In a 16:8 pattern, a person fasts for sixteen hours and only eats during an eight-hour window. In alternate-day fasting, regular eating days alternate with days of significant calorie reduction. All of these approaches revolve around *when* to eat versus *what* to eat in hopes of weight loss or metabolic benefits.

But now there is a good amount of research out there, and here's what it tells us:

- A systematic review and meta-analysis published in *Nutrients* assessed the adverse events associated with intermittent fasting in adults with "overweight" or "obesity" BMI categories. The study identified several potential side effects, including hypoglycemia, dizziness, weakness, fatigue, and headaches. These adverse effects highlight the need for caution and individualized approaches when considering intermittent fasting as a dietary strategy.

- A more concerning study with preliminary data was presented at the EPI|Lifestyle Scientific Sessions in 2024. Researchers looked at a group of 20,000 adults who answered questions about their dietary patterns for the annual National Health and Nutrition Examination Surveys between 2003-2018 and found that individuals practicing the 16:8 intermittent fasting regimen had a 91 percent higher risk of dying from cardiovascular disease compared to those who ate over a typical twelve-to-sixteen-hour window. This increased risk was also observed in individuals with pre-existing cardiovascular conditions. The study suggests that while intermittent fasting may offer short-term benefits, it could pose long-term health risks, particularly for those with heart disease.

- A study published in July 2024 in the *Journal of Trial and Error* examined the effects of intermittent fasting on cognitive functions, mood, and sleep quality over two months. The results indicated no significant improvements in attention, memory, working memory, executive functions, mood, or sleep quality among participants. This suggests that the anticipated cognitive and psychological benefits of intermittent fasting may be overstated, and the practice could have neutral or adverse effects on mental well-being.

- Research published in *Nutrients* reviewed the effects of intermittent fasting on various health parameters. The review highlighted concerns regarding hormonal imbalances, particularly in individuals with existing metabolic conditions. It noted that intermittent fasting could lead to fluctuations in blood glucose levels, which may be detrimental to individuals with diabetes or those at risk of hypoglycemia. Additionally, the review pointed out that fasting without adequate protein intake could result in muscle wasting, emphasizing the need for caution, especially among older adults and those with compromised immune systems.

How did it gain such popularity without scientific backing? Friends, it's because everyone is desperately searching for the solution to a problem that doesn't exist and was created to manipulate us into the never-ending cycle of pursuing weight loss. Anything that promises weight loss has the potential for popularity. The surest, quickest way to gain recognition, and possibly fame and fortune, is to write a weight-loss book with the right marketing.

To be clear, if you are one of the 62 million people (and counting) who has tried some version of IF, you have done nothing wrong. In the 2010s, it was everywhere! What brought so many people into the IF fold was the belief that it provided some sense of control over a body they were made to feel was out of control in terms of weight, size, shape, and even aging. Further, it was an easy concept to understand, even if it's not easy in practice. But what we now know is there are legitimate risks to this approach with none of the intended benefits of long term weight loss.

If your religious or spiritual tradition encourages you to fast for spiritual purposes from time to time and that is in line with your values, then by all means, continue to do so if it brings you closer to your faith and your inner Spirit. This type of fasting won't result in you feeling disconnected from yourself because fasting for spiritual practices isn't about weight loss. It never was.

Spiritual and Physical Hunger

As we talked about in Chapter 2, diet culture completely ignores the needs of the body and disconnects our minds, bodies, and spirits from each other. When that happens, we become intently focused on purposefully ignoring the needs of the body and forget about how that affects our minds and spirits. Think about it. When was the last time you paid attention to your mental health needs, let alone your spiritual health and needs? Diet culture and the distrust we develop about our bodies' innate wisdom (wisdom that's there to keep us alive) starves us of more than just food.

I had the pleasure of speaking with a rabbi about what it means to honor your hunger. She beautifully described it as a "sacred pause" for taking a moment of discernment to ask if this is a mind, body, or spiritual need, which is a practice that's applicable to many areas of life as we move through our days. Sometimes that practice leads to deeper reflection on what it means to consider cravings and longing. And then sometimes it's just not that deep. Sometimes, she said, the answer comes quickly and simply like, "Am I hungry? I just gave birth to twins, so yes, I'm starving!"

At its core, **spiritual hunger is a desire for meaning and purpose** and/or a longing for God. It's a search for understanding and for something that explains the chaos and confusion of the world. There is a deep, spiritual tug beneath the surface that comes from a desire to feel anchored, guided, and lit up by something larger than our routines. As the rabbi put it so well, "Our greater culture can leave us feeling a sense of scarcity. I think spiritual hunger is a desire to cultivate a more expansive, abundant existence for all God's creation. In other words, can we wake up to our spiritual potential and purpose? Can we listen to that faint stirring in our souls that tells us there is more to this material world, more to transactional relationships and more than greedy impulses?"

I suspect anyone who is reading this knows this feeling. I know I do. Honoring your hunger can be a simple and profound principle that applies to both biological and spiritual hunger.

But what if you're really not physically hungry? Do you still need to eat? You can argue this point from different angles, but the answer will be that, regardless of an appetite, yes, you will eventually need to eat.

There are many circumstances that decrease an individual's appetite, such as certain medical conditions, and, medications, grief, depression, and anxiety, to name a few. Yet we logically know that even under these circumstances, we still need to eat to survive. But what if none of those conditions apply, and you've simply gotten used to a busy lifestyle and skipping meals? I would argue that you probably are hungry if you're skipping meals—you've just stopped listening to your hunger cues. (And you may be perpetuating this cycle if there's a secondary benefit of weight loss or weight management because diet culture conditioned you to believe this was desirable.)

Most dieticians agree that outside of sleep, we shouldn't go more than five hours without food, and most suggest eating every three to four hours to maintain blood sugars, energy, and mood. This means that there may be times when your stomach isn't growling yet, but you should still feed it. Our bodies need and deserve that we honor our hunger when we recognize our hunger cues and sometimes even when we don't.

Imagine that you have a quarterly staff meeting tomorrow. It is an all-day meeting from nine to five where you and your team will be sitting in a conference room going over your budget and projections. You wake up at 7:30 a.m. so you can leave by 8:30 a.m. to get there on time. You've been awake for only an hour and are not hungry yet, but they won't be serving lunch until 1 p.m., and you need to stay sharp for this meeting. The recommendation would be to eat something in advance knowing that, even though you're not hungry yet, you will certainly become hungry before 1 p.m.

When I met with my friend and former pastor to talk about this over breakfast, she reminded me about the powerful moment in the story of Elijah from 1 Kings, Chapter 19. Elijah is on the run and is exhausted, afraid, and overwhelmed, and God provides him with food. She reminded me that God was caring for him with food as sustenance and addressed his hunger and fatigue first. God cared for Elijah not just spiritually, but physically and emotionally as well. This story is often used by pastors, therapists, and theologians to emphasize that basic human needs are spiritual matters, too, which is an important reminder for us all.

It's okay to rest.

It's okay to eat.

God meets us there.

All of the incredible things that we wish to accomplish—our hopes and dreams and ambitions and even sometimes just getting through the day—require us to take care of our fundamental needs and adequately nourish our bodies. **Nourishing ourselves helps us become the fully actualized selves the Universe intends us to be.** Even if you're not convinced that the Universe has a stake in your actualization, listening to and honoring our hunger is practicing self-respect and self-compassion. You are deserving of both.

Practice Honoring Your Hunger

As you close this chapter on honoring your hunger, take some time to gently look inward. Consider the messages you absorbed about hunger growing up. Where did these messages come from? Did you learn about hunger from family, culture, and/or religion? How did those teachings shape the way you relate to food today? Did hunger feel like something to trust or something to control? Has fasting ever been part of your religion or culture? Reflect on what your experience has been with emphasis on gaining clarity about your motives. Understanding these roots can help you see how old beliefs still influence your present-day patterns. Imagine hunger as a God-given biological signal, a sacred cue woven into your design. When you view hunger as something intentionally placed within you, not as a flaw or a temptation but as a form of divine communication, what begins to shift inside you?

As you move forward, try setting the goal of noticing your early hunger cues without attempting to change your eating behavior. Pay attention to the subtler signs, too, including irritability, foggy thinking, mood dips, fatigue, and/or that faint sense of hollowness. You may choose to mentally track these or use a journal to see what comes up and if you notice any patterns that may bring you some insights. These gentle signals are part of your body's sacred language. Relearning how to hear them is an act of returning to yourself and can also be thought of as an act of returning to your faith. **Each moment of tuning in becomes a reminder that your body is not an obstacle to overcome but a vessel worthy of care, presence, and trust.**

Chapter Four

Make Peace with Food and Receive It with Grace

For years, I had a sign above my office that read "Life's Short, Eat the Cookie." A coworker gifted it to me because she knew cookies were my favorite thing, but she didn't know about the dark side of my relationship with them. Even though I loved them, I hated them, too. I never bought them because I couldn't trust myself with them. I couldn't just eat one. Heck, I couldn't just eat four. Even if I didn't particularly love the brand or variety, something about the combination of sweet and crunchy was my kryptonite. It's almost strange to think of that now because that relationship has done a 180, and now I wholeheartedly believe in and advocate the "Life's Short, Eat the Cookie" philosophy. But back then, diet culture had me believing that I should feel guilty for loving cookies, guiltier for honoring my cookie hunger and eating them, and guiltiest when I always ate more than one. Working at a hospital at the time, the medical providers would bring me back cookies from the doctors lounge. It was a thing. If a pharmaceutical rep came to our clinic with a tray full of cookies, let's say chocolate chip, oatmeal raisin, sugar and snickerdoodle, I would need to try one of each. It felt compulsory. FOMO.

Perhaps you've experienced something like this. Is there a food that you feel you can't keep in your house? Is there a food you don't trust yourself with? Is there a food that you've determined is off-limits for you? Is there a food that you've deemed as "bad" or "evil" because of the control you believe it has over you? Do you know where these feelings come from? Is it genuinely because those particular foods make you sick? Or is it because you have been told over and over again that you shouldn't like them or eat them?

Poor food. Poor innocent food. It doesn't deserve our vitriol or fear, and it doesn't deserve to be ignored or viewed with disgust. Food has never wanted to fight with us; it has wanted only to nourish us and give us pleasure and satisfaction.

So can we call a truce with food? Can we give up fighting with food and enter into a new healthy relationship that consists of respect and appreciation? If you've already started the process of rejecting diet culture and agree with and practice honoring your hunger, this is easier. Even if you haven't started rejecting diet culture, I would still encourage you to try honoring your hunger without judgment, and see how you feel. Know that God and the Universe want this peaceful relationship for you, too. This is what the principle of making peace with your food is about: moving away from viewing food as the enemy and instead looking at it as the blessing it was and is always meant to be.

For the Love of God and Potatoes: How Food Becomes Enemy #1

Have you ever been at a table where someone said a blessing before the meal? Even if this isn't part of your typical routine, my guess is you've experienced it at least once, perhaps at a friend's house or at a Christmas Eve party where Uncle Tony gave a wine-slurred speech before carving the turkey. Whether you've heard a blessing before a meal once or a thousand times, they all have one thing in common: They give thanks for the food itself. And in that moment, this seems to be a concept everyone can get behind. We are grateful for the food, for Aunt Edna's famous rice-crispy-encrusted fried chicken and Grandmom's homemade apple pie. If we are lucky, we smile and enjoy the bounty at the table before us.

In my family, a Morse holiday feast is something to behold. There is usually an extra-long table where every inch is covered with trays of food and bottles of drink. (My cousin actually had her extra long table custom-made, and it's enormous.) My father always exclaims, "So much food!" as if he's surprised; meanwhile, he always arrives at the party with his hands full of contributions to the festivities. And the only thing louder than the yummy "mmmmm" sounds is the laughter. We eat. We laugh. We repeat. It's wonderful and life-giving. **This is what God wants for us. He wants us to enjoy food, even in its abundance.**

But then the meal slows down, and you start to hear the familiar sounds of, "Ugh I'm so full, I feel disgusting," or, "I can't believe I ate so much, I couldn't eat another bite," or at its worst, "Guess I'm not eating anything the rest of the weekend." How quickly it changes from smiles, joy, and gratitude back to thinking of food as the enemy!

In their fourth edition of *Intuitive Eating: A Revolutionary Anti-Diet Approach,* Evelyn Tribole and Elyse Resch describe five potential fears that get in the way of making peace with food: won't stop eating, pseudo permission, self-fulfilling prophecy, becoming unhealthy, lack of self-trust. I'll discuss each of the five below, but of them, I hear the first fear most frequently: "I won't stop eating." So many people have been restricting for so long and have created so many rules that they are truly afraid that eliminating said rules will lead to a never-ending binge. (This does differ from a professionally diagnosed condition such as binge eating disorder.) In the interest of full transparency, there is partial truth to this. They may not be able to stop eating *at first.* And that "at first" piece is a critical difference. There is absolutely a possibility that you may behave like a kid in a candy store at first, but this is a short-term, temporary phase, a backlash to the psychological deprivation of dieting. But your body and your cravings will adjust once your brain and body realize that those restrictions are no longer in effect. For most people, it happens much sooner than they think.

Psychological deprivation during dieting refers to the mental and emotional experience of being restricted. For example, think of all your self-imposed food rules, which often come from the perception that certain foods are off-limits and/or that eating must be tightly controlled. Yet, after you no longer deem those foods as off-limit, the desire for them actually diminishes.

Not convinced? Imagine this. Think of the food that feels the scariest to you, the one you feel you have no control over and therefore should never allow it into your home. Let's name it *Tasty X* for this example. Tasty X is your favorite treat. You think it is the most delicious treat you've ever had, and you feel helpless against it.

Now let's imagine that you've just won a sweepstakes, and the prize is a lifetime supply of Tasty X. Tomorrow, a truck will deliver five thousand boxes of Tasty X to your doorstep. Will you tear into the first box? Probably! Maybe even the second one. But will you eat all five thousand boxes in one sitting? Of course not. Why? Because one, you will no longer feel the pull of your desire as you have an endless supply, and two, you will start to feel pretty sick pretty fast.

This is the power of psychological deprivation. When you deprive yourself of a particular food, when your brain believes that thing is now scarce, you will want it more, but when you allow yourself to have it, you decrease the power it has over you. It's honestly that simple. I didn't say it was easy, but it is simple.

Psychological scarcity, hand in hand with arbitrary food rules, can also lead to the Binge-Restrict Food Cycle, or BRFC for short. The BRFC describes the pattern that many of us have fallen victim to multiple times. It looks like this: Tracey read that potatoes aren't good for us. Instead of looking for the research backing up this claim, she became caught up in the diet culture reasoning that potatoes could be blamed for an inability to lose weight. Tracey, having felt frustrated for years about not being able to consistently keep weight off, hoped that she may have finally found the reason. She decided to cut out all potatoes from her diet, even though she only ate them about once a week anyway.

A few days later, she was constantly thinking about potatoes and the many mouth-watering, delicious ways to eat them: baked potatoes, hash browns, home fries, roasted potatoes, gnocchi, pierogies, au gratin potatoes, scalloped potatoes, potato chips, mashed potatoes, dumplings, twice-baked potatoes, potato skins, tater tots, and of course French fries! How had she never realized this before?

A couple weeks later, Tracey found herself actually dreaming of potatoes. Not long after her first potato-filled dream, she went to a steakhouse with some friends and saw on the menu that you could get *four* different types of potatoes. What was she to do? She hadn't realized how much she actually liked potatoes until she stopped eating them. In a moment of panic and exhilaration, Tracey ordered all four kinds of potatoes and ravenously ate every bite of them. It happened so fast that she had no idea what she was doing. It was like an out-of-body experience. But after eating them, not only was she very physically uncomfortable, she also felt guilty and ashamed. Of course, she placed the blame for her physical and emotional discomfort on our poor friend the potato, and she again vowed to restrict them the very next day.

And around and around we go. That's the BRFC.

(**If there was ever a gift in the form of food, it is the potato.** Please do your bodies, minds, and souls the favor of showing them the respect, enjoyment, and the appreciation they deserve.

In fact, let's take a moment. Okay, moment over. Moving on . . . .)

Perhaps it's not just one specific food or food group that you've decided to restrict. Perhaps it's an overall reduction in food and calories. Here's what we know: The number one predictor of a binge episode is hunger. The majority of people who experience binge episodes experience them in the evening, and it isn't hard to guess why. They have been restricting all day, resulting in undereating, and their intense feelings of hunger then result in a binge episode. And what is truly the most addictive food? Perhaps you've guessed it by now. **The most addictive food on the planet is the one you restrict.** But as you just learned, giving yourself permission to eat said addictive food lessens, and eventually eliminates, its power over you. (Note: Having a binge episode does not necessarily meet criteria for binge-eating disorder. Only a licensed mental health professional can make this diagnosis.)

Addressing another fear that Evelyn and Elyse highlight is the pseudo-permission: "I've tried it before." Those of us working in the field of disordered eating find this is often a barrier. People tell us that they've tried allowing themselves to eat the forbidden foods in the past, but they always end up overeating. What they're missing is that the barrier is actually the way they view food as "forbidden" in the first place. They typically haven't tried this free-wheeling food permission before because they believe they shouldn't be eating food they consider "bad" or "unhealthy." (That's the diet mentality we dismantled in Chapter 2.) Maybe they were doing their best in trying to commit to a new behavior, but they had little chance of success because their minds were still swept up in said diet mentality.

A third fear is the self-fulfilling prophecy. This is when a person predicts they will have a sequence of events unfold, which results in them manifesting the very outcome they were afraid would happen. For example, if I allow myself to have a piece of chocolate and then obsessively fear that this creates an inability to stop eating the chocolate, that anxiety and worrying may result in overeating the chocolate. Fortunately, unconditional permission to eat is not a lone skill. It exists as part of the comprehensive philosophical model of intuitive eating that can help in preventing these self-fulfilling prophecies.

Next is the fear that "I won't eat healthfully." Similar to the first fear we discussed of being unable to stop eating, there is a reasonable chance that you will first go after the foods you previously deemed "bad" or "unhealthy." Why wouldn't you? Let's say you ate in the same restaurant for a month, and there were only two items on the menu: a green salad and a fruit salad. Then one day, there is a cheeseburger with fries. Of course you will choose the new food item! The same logic applies that after limiting your eating world to only "healthy foods." You may likely choose other options. However, you will quickly find that your body will not want that cheeseburger and fries every day, either. If that were to become the only item on the menu, you would soon get sick of it as well. **The more you learn to listen intuitively, the wider your eating circle becomes.**

The last fear some people face is a lack of self-trust. This fear could really be the overarching title of the ones we've already reviewed. At its core, intuitive eating isn't just about food choices; it's about trusting your body's signals and learning to listen without judgment. When someone has a lack of self-trust, it impacts every aspect of their relationship with food, their body, and their emotional well-being. Diet culture is built on the idea that there is a "perfect" way to eat. When people internalize this culture, they stop trusting themselves and instead rely on external rules about what, when, and how much to eat. Any deviation from the "ideal" is seen as failure.

A lack of self-trust often goes hand in hand with a lack of self-compassion. If a person doesn't trust themselves, they may be overly critical of their own food choices or body, perpetuating feelings of unworthiness. **Without self-compassion, it's hard to heal from the past or build trust with oneself.** Overcoming this barrier requires a mindset shift from external control to internal trust, and it can be a profound journey of healing—not just with food, but with the self. And like anything else, it takes practice.

If we return to our Tasty X example, even if some of the above fears were present initially, I suspect two things. First, the behaviors of those fears would be very short term, and second, if the following year you won another contest, this time with a lifetime supply of Tasty Y, there may be little to no evidence of those fear behaviors being present at all.

Permission for Peace

One of the most beautiful but complex aspects of intuitive eating is the concept of giving yourself unconditional permission to eat. Unconditional permission to eat is exactly what it sounds like: You eat what you want. You allow yourself to eat any and all foods because there are no longer any "good" or "bad" foods. You eat when you are hungry because you no longer have any rules about such things, and you are now able to listen to your body's needs.

It's not "time" for lunch yet, but you're already hungry? Eat.

You just ate two hours ago, but you're hungry again? Eat.

That forbidden food you feel you have no control over was just offered to you, and it looks delicious? Eat.

No one embodies this better than Joey Tribbiani, the beloved character from the iconic sitcom *Friends,* played by Matt LeBlanc. Joey allows himself unconditional permission to eat. Never is this more clear than the Thanksgiving episode where Rachel Green (another beloved character played by Jennifer Aniston) attempts to make dessert for her friends. However, she makes the terrible mistake of accidentally blending two recipes into one. She makes an English trifle, her intended dessert, but erroneously adds the ingredients of a shepherd's pie. Thus, she layers ladyfingers, jam, homemade custard, raspberries, more ladyfingers, then beef sautéed with peas and onions, then a little more custard, then bananas, and finally whipped cream on top.

As her friends look on in both confusion and disbelief, they decide they don't want to hurt her feelings and eat it anyway. Except for dear Joey, all of the friends at the table can get only one bite down and then make an excuse to leave. When one of the friends states in disgust, "This tastes like feet," Joey takes yet another bite. "What's not to like?" he says as he dives in again for another taste. "Custard good. Jam good. Meat gooooood."

Maybe we don't all need to allow ourselves to eat beef in our desserts, but we can open the door to more possibilities and less restrictions. And for me that means cookies!

This concept of making peace with food and giving myself permission to eat and enjoy it has been one of the most life-changing elements for me within the intuitive eating model. Nothing is off limits because nothing is forbidden. Nothing is avoided because nothing is "bad." Food is equal. Food is neutral. And (gratefully) food is accessible.

Remember my secret love-hate relationship with cookies? With this tenet of intuitive eating, I was able to break the cycle of psychological deprivation that had kept its hold over me and now I can eat only one cookie, if I want. But I can also eat four or more, if I want. That's the point: It's my choice.

What's been fascinating and completely freeing is that there is no longer any food I feel I have no control over, including cookies. Because I allow myself to have something sweet whenever I want, I no longer crave sweets and don't feel any pull or desire to have a cookie if I'm not in the mood. I've even discovered there are several kinds I don't even really like! Most store-bought cookies I would have compulsively eaten in the past now taste dry and too sweet for me. That said, it's rare I'll turn down someone's homemade cookies, and I do enjoy Oreos and Pepperidge Farm Double Chocolate Milanos. But now they'll last a week or two in my house instead of only two hours.

In 2007, researchers Esther Jansen, Sandra Mulkens, and Anita

Jansen conducted a study in which they provided children with M&Ms but told the kids they were not allowed to eat the red ones. Adults were present in the room, and so the children complied with the rule, for the most part. However, as soon as the rule was lifted and they could eat any color candy they wanted, guess which one they all went after? The red ones, of course! It didn't matter that they all tasted the same. It didn't matter that prior to the experiment, it would have been unlikely they all chose red as their favorite. But once it was off limits and forbidden, it became more desirable.

This is true for all of us: when something is "off limits" for arbitrary reasons, it becomes the focus of our desire. However, the converse is also true: **Once you give yourself full and complete, unconditional permission to eat, the flip switches in your brain, and you no longer feel deprived.** The excitement and pull diminishes so you will no longer feel the need to overindulge unless you choose to, and there is so much freedom in that. This is how I made peace with cookies. This is how you can make peace with any food.

Embracing a Heart of Peace and Joy

One year, at the start of Diwali, I attended a networking event for local clinicians where they served delicious Indian food and taught us about this festival of lights. Diwali is a joyful, multi-day celebration that symbolizes the victory of light over darkness, good over evil, and knowledge over ignorance. The organizer of the event was both a registered dietician and a licensed therapist, a rare and brilliant combination. During the event, I had the opportunity to thank her for organizing it and shared how much I enjoyed myself and learning about her culture. She must have believed my sincerity because she promptly invited me to her home the following weekend for a traditional Diwali party complete with food and dancing. I couldn't wait.

Two days before the party, I found myself at an annual Rotary Club fundraiser called Pours for Polio. My husband is very active in the local rotary club, which is a volunteer-based service organization, and we had been several times before this. It was held at a local bar known for their live music and a diverse selection of beers. After greeting our friends, we found ourselves standing near a couple he didn't recognize. Being the enthusiastic extrovert I am, I took my very introverted husband over to introduce ourselves, and well, we were meant to meet this couple. Clearly the Universe had orchestrated this meeting. I had so many things in common with the wife, and my husband so many things in common with her husband. She and I were both yoga teachers, both mindfulness practitioners, both vegetarians, both writers, and both very eager to make new friends. It was an instant connection.

At one point during our lively conversation, we started talking about the season of Diwali. I mentioned I was going to my first Diwali party. The wife asked me what I was wearing, and I said I was advised to wear something colorful. She said, "Come to my home tomorrow, I will give you something appropriate to wear."

I declined her invitation out of politeness while secretly hoping she would insist.

And thank goodness she did.

"We're nearly the same size. I have so many. Please come to our home. We would love to have you."

My husband had also enjoyed his conversation so much that we agreed.

The next morning, we drove twenty minutes to their beautiful home and were instantly treated like family who has been there a million times. In less than five minutes, they were feeding us. The husband grew giant Indian squash in his garden, and I mean giant. The wife made *halwa,* a sweet Indian squash pudding popular during Diwali festivals. It was delicious. This is how we show our hearts: with food and kindness, and then more food.

After we sat chitchatting and eating for a while, she brought me into another room where she had laid out four beautiful, traditional Indian outfits. She assured me they were all perfect for a Diwali party. I enjoyed what I can only describe as a movie montage moment as I tried on each outfit and came out to the living room to smile and twirl, letting my host's mother—who did not speak a word of English—tell me how lovely I looked. At least that's what I was told.

Once I'd selected my favorite dress (the bright, hot-pink one, of course), I asked if there was a special place to do the dry cleaning for such an ornate piece of clothing before returning to her. She said absolutely not, she had a ton of dresses, and it would give her joy to let me keep one. I was struck with this woman's generosity and love for someone she'd only just met. She fed me and dressed me, and it was a beautiful day.

Imagine if she and I had been immersed in diet culture. For starters, we may never have even met because many people who are deep in the clutches of diet culture avoid social situations. But even if we had met, perhaps we would've been too uncomfortable in our own skin to even put ourselves out there to let a friendship blossom. I may have still found my way to her home, but what if she didn't feed me because she didn't want to have anything sweet herself? What if I had declined because I was afraid of how much sugar or calories might be in it? Or what if when I was trying on these gorgeous dresses, I was self-conscious and not wanting to show anyone how I looked and therefore missed my montage moment? Even worse, what if I compared my body to hers, thereby drawing an imaginary line between us? Fortunately, this wasn't the case at all. Not even for a moment, and I was able to enjoy a meaningful connection and receive food and generosity with grace.

Later that weekend, I had an amazing time at the Diwali party. Feasting, dancing, talking, and repeat. As soon as I entered the home of my colleague, I was hit with the mouthwatering aroma of food. I quickly found the hostess who, in the same breath of welcoming me to her home, handed me a drink with my name written on the cup. She informed me it was limeade, fresh mint, and cumin, a combination I never would've tried elsewhere or on my own. Of course, it was wonderful.

I spent the next few minutes being introduced to some other women before being ushered to the table where a bountiful feast was beautifully laid out. There must have been a dozen different trays on the table, not including the dessert table on the other side of the kitchen. I needed to try a bite of everything. And I did with pleasure and no guilt. My plate was quite full when I found my seat on the couch with a number of women gorgeously dressed in bright and sparkly saris.

I don't recall everything I tried, but I do remember my favorites: the *malai kofta,* which is a soft deep-fried potato/paneer dumpling in a creamy tomato-based sauce; the cabbage carrot *sambharo,* which is a stir-fry with cabbage, carrot, and bell pepper; and then the samosas, a pastry stuffed with savory mixed vegetables. For dessert, I had the *galub jamun* almond cake, an almond-flour cake flavored with cardamom and soaked in saffron and rose syrup. I also had *mohanthal,* an Indian sweet made from besan flour, sugar syrup, ghee and flavored with cardamom. I love Indian food. This was a feast to write about. Literally.

Following the meal, our host invited her guests into her garage where she had created a dance floor. We were going to learn a traditional dance common at Diwali parties that involved *dandiyas,* or colorful sticks, that you rhythmically strike together during the steps of the dance. The music was lively, the guests were all smiles, and our host was beaming. My heart and soul were full.

Before we left, our host gave a little speech. Not only did she thank us for coming and helping her make a new beautiful memory for her home, she also shared how important it is that we share our cultures with one another. We can share our hearts and our food and open up our homes to one another. She was grateful we shared in the feast and festivities of Diwali with her. This is what receiving food with grace can look like. This is how we heal our relationship with food.

Our Birthright: Feasting with Gladness

"Go, eat your food with gladness, drink your wine with a joyful heart, for God has already approved what you do." (Ecclesiastes 9:7) I love this verse. It encourages people to enjoy life, specifically food and drink, without guilt. These are not frivolous pleasures; they are divine blessings. This isn't indulgence, it's reverence. Eat with gladness. Drink with joy. God gives us this spiritual invitation. When we're stuck in diet culture or following strict, non-medically advised food rules or ignoring our hunger, we miss these opportunities for connection.

We see references to a positive association with food throughout the world. **In nearly every major religion, feasting is a way to honor the divine, celebrate community, mark holy times, and express gratitude.** It is a sacred and meaningful practice. Eating and enjoying God's creation is a form of worship.

In the Christian faith, the heavenly banquet represents the eternal joyful communion with God where there is no hunger, no exclusion, and no sorrow; there is only abundance, belonging, and peace. Buddhism, typically known for its simplistic lifestyle, still participates in communal feasts for various celebrations. And the many faith traditions that participate in fasting oftentimes break the fast with a celebratory feast. In the Islam faith, the feast comes at the end of Ramadan. It's known as the Festival of Breaking the Fast, and it's a day of joy, gratitude, renewal, and reconnection with God, family, and community.

If you don't currently follow any traditional faith tradition, allow me to provide a more secular example. There is a scene in the first Harry Potter movie (yes I am a nerd and love fantasy books and films) where Harry and his friends sit down in the great hall for the first time, and Professor Dumbledore says, "Let the feast begin!" All of a sudden, the previously bare tables are magically covered with what appears to be an endless bounty of a variety of different kinds of food. The eyes of the children are wide with wonder, excitement, and disbelief. They have no hesitation digging in with both hands. They receive it fully with excitement, curiosity, and freedom. There's no internal debate about what's "good" or "bad," no calorie counting, no guilt. Just pure presence and delight in the moment.

Like sacred feasts across spiritual traditions, feasting in general reflects a deep truth that we are meant to receive nourishment with gratitude and celebration, not fear. The feast reminds us that food is not just fuel, but also magic, connection, and joy. Can you remember a time in your own life when that was the case and you were excited about food? In that moment, food is an incredible blessing.

My hope is that there is a part of you right now, even a small part, that is starting to see the possibility of having a wildly different relationship with food and maybe even the potential and value of making peace with it. Celebrate this! It is a brave and difficult thing to open ourselves up to different perspectives, especially as adults.

However, we still have work to do. If we were sitting together right now, I suspect you would have dozens of questions for me, many of which would start with "But what about…" That's great! Questions are normal. But it's important to know why those questions are coming up and where they're coming from, which is why the next chapter is about the food police.

Practice Making Peace with Food

As you prepare to step more fully into making peace with food, it can help to look back on the moments when eating felt joyful, connective, or even sacred. When was the last time eating felt like this? Think of the meals that stand out in your memory. Perhaps they were celebrations where the only thing louder than the clanking of dishes was the cackling of laughter. Or maybe they were cultural feasts that reminded you of where you come from. In those moments, something in you softened, and you allowed yourself to let go. **Food was no longer an enemy to control but a bridge to belonging.** Let yourself remember what shifted inside you when nourishment felt like an expression of love instead of a test you were supposed to pass, even if it only happened once. Try to remember what that felt like and share the story with someone you trust or write it down in your journal.

To go even further in your journey, choose one food you have labeled as forbidden or off limits and gently allow it back into your home. No conditions, no negotiations, simply permission. I know this may be scary. I get it. Remember the five fears? Flip back to page 63 and re-read that section for encouragement whenever you need it. If I'm being honest with you, it may not go the way you hope it will at first. But let this be an experiment. Let this be a practice in trust, both in your body and in the idea that you were never meant to live in fear of the things that are meant to nourish you. You can also take a small step toward connection by saying yes to one food-centered experience this week. Share a meal with someone you love, accept an invitation, bake alongside a friend, or try a recipe from a culture different from your own. These simple acts have a way of opening the heart. In embracing them, you're not just making peace with food, you're opening yourself to community, curiosity, and the sacredness woven into everyday nourishment.

Chapter Five

Challenge the Food Police and Quiet the Inner Critic

Imagine you're pushing your cart through the grocery store to pick up a few ingredients for dinner. You have a variety of things in the basket: a couple of zucchini, an onion, spaghetti noodles, and a jar of sauce. As you stand in the frozen food aisle debating whether you want breadsticks or garlic bread, the customer next to you reaches into your cart and pulls out the jar of sauce.

"This has too much sugar in it … for *you,*" they say, and walk away, jar of sauce in hand.

What would you do?

One of my favorite authors and activists, Aubrey Gordon, wrote about these kinds of experiences in her must-read book *What We Don't Talk About When We Talk About Fat.*

We've all grown up around bullies and are familiar with name calling, the silent treatment, stealing, pushing someone down, teasing, mocking, pranking, spreading rumors, and so on, but I've never encountered someone removing a food item from my grocery cart. How did we get here? In what world does someone think that's okay?

My sincere hope is that someone who polices other people's food choices believes they are being helpful and not deliberately cruel. However, not only is it cruel, but research reports that being a victim of weight stigma actually puts an individual at higher risk for health problems, including higher blood pressure, higher cortisol levels, higher blood sugar levels, and higher depression and anxiety symptoms. It also encourages and justifies the cruelty of our inner food police, the subject of this principle: challenge the food police.

The food police live deep in our psyche where we determine who we are, who we want to be, how we identify ourselves, and how we believe we ought to behave. And if we're really honest with ourselves, most of us have a much stricter inner voice, or full-on police force, than what we typically experience from others. This inner policing does not serve and protect our health at all. Instead, it draws us away from the sacred relationship we are meant to have with our bodies. **Anything that governs the body through shame rather than love cannot be a path to true health or spiritual wholeness.**

Passing Down the Food Police from Generation to Generation

How many times have you beaten yourself up for eating something you feel you shouldn't have? How many times have you felt guilty about eating "too much" or shame around clothes feeling too tight? Have you been disgusted with yourself over a perceived sense of failure around willpower?

In the words of the talented pop star Demi Lovato, "I'm guilty 'bout everything that I eat (every single thing) / Feelin' myself is a felony / Jedi level sabotage / Voices in my head make up my entourage." Sound familiar?

Where did this voice come from? Did it come from your family? Did it come from advertisements and models? Did it come from social media and influencers? Did it come from weight loss companies? Maybe several of these sources? Maybe all of them?

When my niece was in kindergarten, she was already getting messages at school about what kinds of snacks were good and bad, healthy and unhealthy. Yes, it starts that early. In fact, because of language like this, all of it from diet culture, children as young as four years old learn to understand the word "fat" as an insult. Here's a scary statistic: At ages six to ten, girls start to worry about their weight, and by age fourteen, 60 percent to 70 percent are trying to lose weight.

This isn't rocket science right? Parents don't want their children to suffer. The adults who have confided in me that they struggle with the fight against diet culture confidently say they do not want that struggle for their children. At the same time, I have seen countless examples, both professionally and personally, of parents taking a "do what I say, not what I do" attitude when it comes to dieting and their relationship with food because they are unable to silence the voice of their own inner food police. They will genuinely tell their children to enjoy the piece of birthday cake while not allowing themselves to partake. They tell their children with heartfelt sincerity that they are beautiful just the way they are while secretly hating their own bodies. They will allow their kids to have a snack before bed when they say they're hungry, but then ignore their own hunger cues and tell themselves they can't.

The voice of the food police is loud and eager, and it's successful at diminishing our sense of self because diet culture rewards and celebrates this voice. Diet culture is the food police cheerleader championing the rules, restrictions, and black-and-white thinking. **Should you ever start to think outside of this confining box, the food police are ever ready to throw counter-arguments your way with a hefty side of guilt and shame.**

The food police voice is easy to recognize once you become

aware of it. It is strict, often unkind, and usually has a berating tone. Here are some examples:

- *I shouldn't have eaten that cupcake; it has too many calories.*
- *I'm such a failure for stopping for fast food.*
- *It's after 7 p.m. and I'm hungry, but I can't eat anything this late.*
- *I can't have chips in the house; I have no control when they are around.*
- *I ate too much at lunch so I shouldn't eat dinner.*
- *I'll have to workout an extra thirty minutes at the gym later to burn this off*
- *I just had breakfast. How am I already hungry again?*
- *Good job saying no to that slice of birthday cake.*
- *I deserve to feel sick; I ate too much.*
- *I cheated on my diet again. I have no willpower.*

You get the gist. If you're entrenched in diet culture, you could come up with many more, I'm sure. Every time we listen to the food police, every time we give into that horrible voice, we strengthen it. We perpetuate diet culture by ignoring our hunger or desire for connection to ourselves and others.

A True Psychological Thriller

For about six months, I lived in the panhandle of Florida in a town called Chattahoochee. I was completing an internship program at Florida State Hospital and working with forensic psychiatric patients. I was deeply invested in learning and growing as a clinician, but outside of work, there really wasn't too much to do in the small rural area. There was a Piggly Wiggly grocery store, a Dairy Queen, and a local soul-food restaurant. Despite the lack of a social scene, I really enjoyed my internship and learned a lot. But when I returned home to New Jersey, instead of comments about how I'd grown professionally, there were suddenly frequent comments about the change in my body size and shape from my time away.

I know it may not seem possible, but I truly hadn't noticed. I was young, learning to be an independent adult, and finding my way in a new career. Thoughts about my body just weren't top of mind for me. That is, until everyone else noticed started making comments, both subtle and not-so-subtle.

One of the first things I noticed after hearing negative things about my body was an almost instant and significant shift in my mindset from self-security to obsessively comparing myself to every other female in my life and even strangers on the street. When I realized some other women my age had much thinner body types and were much more physically desirable, the noise in my head became so loud at times that it pushed all other (more useful) thoughts out of my mind.

So I did what most people have done for generations: I went on a diet. That first diet changed everything for me. I was one of over a million people attending Weight Watchers meetings in the early 2000s. Their point system required me to be on a very low-calorie, restrictive diet.

As you can imagine, drastically cutting my calories along with daily aerobics resulted in "successful" weigh-ins each week at the meetings. I dropped a lot of weight fast. I was a success story! I even earned Lifetime Member status because I hit my "goal weight." But that was only what happened on the outside.

On the inside, my thoughts had become obsessive. Food wasn't food anymore; food was points. *How many points can I have for lunch? I'm going out later. Do I have enough points in the day? Oh, I can't have too many points. Oh, that's safe to eat, that's only a few points.* In just a matter of weeks, my brain was flooded with this noise, which continued for years. Eventually I stopped going to Weight Watchers and tried a dozen other diets over the next decade. The noise in my head was incessant. *Don't eat that. That has too many calories. That has too much fat. That has too much sugar. You can't have that you didn't exercise today. You need to do at least an hour of cardio to work that off. You can't eat dinner you ate too much for lunch. You can't eat breakfast you had too much for dinner last night. You have to be really good today. You were so bad this weekend.* It wasn't until many years later I had a name for it: the food police.

The sad part is that I didn't start out with food police in my head. None of us do. We're not born with a food-police part of the brain. Rather, my food police, and those of others, is implanted in our psyches through offhand comments born of diet culture.

Tuning In to Your Inner Voice

What if we didn't have food police at all? What if we could take the guidance we give our children and turn it back on ourselves? What if we could turn the language of the food police around and transform it into a food cheerleader?

- *Good job saying yes to that slice of birthday cake. It feels good to celebrate with those I love.*
- *I want to work out an extra thirty minutes at the gym today to build muscle faster because I love feeling strong. Then I'll have a great meal just because.*
- *I feel sick. I ate too much. It happens. Next time I'll save some of it so I can enjoy it again later. But for now, I'll drink some peppermint tea to soothe my stomach.*

- *I didn't eat enough at lunch, so it was good I stopped for some fast food. Otherwise I'd be too hangry to concentrate at my daughter's swim meet.*

What if we could break the cycle of disordered eating that gets passed down and perpetuated and instead teach children how to have a healthy relationship with food and their bodies? It won't always be easy, but it would be worth it to save the next generation from hearing the food police in their own minds. (Side note: If you're a parent and are interested in learning more about specific parenting strategies, I highly recommend *How to Raise an Intuitive Eater* by Sumner Brooks and Amee Severson.)

According to the founders of intuitive eating and several of my colleagues, **the ultimate weapon against the food police is to become compassionately self-aware of these thoughts.** There are many different therapeutic models that therapists might employ when working with a client in this pursuit. Some models work toward challenging these thoughts, while other models may work on accepting and detaching from them. As a therapist, I have been trained in many therapeutic models. However, later in my career, I discovered one called Acceptance and Commitment Therapy.

Acceptance and Commitment Therapy, otherwise known as ACT, is a therapeutic model born from older behavioral models such as Cognitive Behavioral Therapy (CBT). As an ACT practitioner, I assist individuals in learning how to listen internally and honor what is truly important to them with intention. This is one of the six principles of ACT known as "values," or the qualities you most want to embody. To develop this ability to listen internally, an individual learns and practices the six core principles of ACT with the goal of cultivating psychological flexibility, one of the most beautiful parts of ACT. These six principles are:

- Staying present in the moment

- Accepting our thoughts and feelings versus avoiding or making attempts to change them
- "Unhooking" from those unhelpful thoughts (a defusion skill) so that the thoughts have less power and control
- Creating a "self as-context," separating ourselves from internalizing our thoughts and feelings and having a more fluid, detached perception of self
- Looking to our values for direction and purpose
- Taking committed action towards building the life you want and that is consistent with your values.

Essentially, ACT helps people live more authentically by tuning in to their inner experience. Tuning into this inner experience versus tuning into the food police can be life changing. We can accept that we hear the food police but remember that we are not defined by it. We also learn to remember our values and what is really most important to us so we can make decisions based on those values instead of basing our decisions on the taunts, criticisms, and deceptions of the food police.

One of the key elements in dismantling the food police noise is to notice when it arises. This is actually easier said than done, especially if you've lived with the food police in your mind for decades. It starts with slowing down and paying attention to your thoughts as they relate to food. Then, most importantly, you approach those thoughts with curiosity and kindness. You can't quiet the rigidity and negativity of the food police with criticism and judgment. Instead, notice that the food police thoughts are present and that there are a variety of ways to address them. You might reflect on the source and where the idea came from. Is it something you heard from someone? You might also challenge the truth of the thought. For example, if the food police are telling you there is too much sugar in the juicy mango you're eyeing at the grocery store, you can silence them with some nutritional facts, such as mangos are very nutrient dense, high in vitamins C, A, and B9, and high in fiber and antioxidants. I find both techniques highly effective.

Perhaps my favorite, though, is to use more of an ACT approach and simply accept that these thoughts and feelings come and go like all thoughts and feelings come and go as part of the human experience. Another ACT defusion skill is called "Naming the Story." This labels the stories the mind tells in an effort to distance yourself from them so they lose their power and emphasis. The thought, "There's too much fat in that buttercream icing" might pop up, and I can respond with, "Ah, there's the food police voice again." In naming this as a food police story, it creates a pause or a break in the sequence of thought to behavior. It separates me from my mind and shifts the relationship I have with those thoughts. Without any shame or self-criticism, it supports the effort that thoughts do not need to dictate behavior. You can really personalize this as well for whatever thoughts the food police shout at you that feel so authoritative. For example, if you find that you restrict certain foods because those foods are "bad," that could become "This is the good versus bad story. Those silly food police."

For our purposes in this chapter, let's consider an additional method (similar to ACT): keep listening internally but change the channel. **Turn off the noise of the food police, change the dial, and turn up the volume on your inner voice.** The inner voice can mean many things to many people. For some, it may mean your inner wisdom, your conscience, or your truest self. It may mean our ability to apply reason and integrity.

For some, listening to our inner voice can be a deeply spiritual experience that many people believe connects them to a higher power. In Christianity, it's often referred to as the Holy Spirit speaking within us. In Islam, it may be the *fitrah,* the innate disposition towards God. In Eastern philosophies like Buddhism or Hinduism, it might be seen as the *atman* (true self) or inner guru. In New Age or metaphysical beliefs, the inner voice might be the higher self, a more evolved or spiritually connected part of us. In all of these systems, listening to that voice is seen as opening ourselves to something greater than our ego, something that transcends the immediate and the superficial.

Think about it. Can you recall an experience when you listened to your inner voice? Did you feel a sense of purpose or a deep knowing? Many people describe these moments as feeling "guided" or "held" by something greater than themselves. When we act in accordance with our inner voice, we feel more authentic. We are being true to ourselves and our spiritual path. That integrity can deepen our relationship with a higher power because we're no longer just following external rules. We are living from a place of deep inner truth.

As we get better at listening to our inner voice, we often notice that it does not always point us toward the path of least resistance. Instead, it may be truth over convenience and/or courage over comfort. This moral clarity is often interpreted as being in alignment with a higher power's will, nature, or universal laws (like karma, dharma, or divine order). **Whether you believe in God, the Universe, or simply the power of the human soul, your inner voice can be a sacred bridge, a meeting place between the human self and the divine.**

There's a story in the Bible where Jesus is speaking to a crowd after a confrontation with those who criticized his disciples for eating without ceremonially washing their hands. This was a Jewish purity tradition supporting ritual cleanliness. Jesus responded to the criticism by calling out the hypocrisy of focusing on outer behaviors such as food laws and rituals while neglecting the greater purpose. "Don't you see that nothing that enters a person from the outside can defile them? ... It doesn't go into their heart but into their stomach, and then out of the body. What comes out of a person is what defiles them." (Mark 7:18–20) He declares all foods clean and teaches that real defilement isn't about food or rituals but our thoughts, words, and actions. In doing so, Jesus directly dismantles the labeling of food as "good" or "bad" and dismisses any assigned moral value. He calls people back to heart-centered faith that values mercy, humility, and love over appearance or rule-following. And he challenges those enforcing purity rules, much like we're called to challenge the inner and cultural "food police."

The apostle Paul expands on Jesus's teaching with, "Let not the one who eats despise the one who abstains, and let not the one who abstains pass judgment on the one who eats, for God has welcomed him. Who are you to pass judgment on the servant of another? It is before his own master that he stands or falls." (Romans 14:1–4) Jesus urges believers to focus on unity in love rather than superiority based on rules or restrictions. Our faith is not measured by our diets and whether someone follows a plant-based lifestyle, avoids processed foods, or enjoys fast food; what matters most is the heart, not the menu.

Our hearts know not to listen to the food police. We would never say to someone else the things we say to ourselves. As practitioners of intuitive eating, we would never tell someone we love and care for that they should feel shame or guilt about eating or that they are undeserving of taking care of their bodies with the nourishment and enjoyment of food.

We absolutely can stop doing this to ourselves. When the food police inevitably show up, we can tell it to move on. We can accept the thoughts while changing our relationship to them. We can listen to our inner wisdom or inner voice and follow the path aligned with our values. You deserve better. You deserve peace, and you deserve love. And you deserve to enjoy the wonderful satisfaction of food.

Practice Challenging the Food Police

It can be powerful to pause and reflect on the voices that have shaped your own relationship with food. Sometimes it echoes a parent's worries, a doctor's warnings, cultural ideals, religious expectations, or the endless commentary of the media. Take a moment to notice which judgments show up most often and what kind of tone they carry. Naming these influences helps you recognize that these messages were learned and are not inherent truths.

Next, imagine someone you love deeply struggling with food or body concerns. Picture their face and think about their humanity. Conjure up everything you love about them. What would you say to them if they felt shame and guilt about eating? What would be your actual words to them? Most people respond with compassion, reassurance, and love, yet those same gentle words rarely find their way inward. However, there is good news here. Your ability to find those gentle words for another shows the spiritual truth that compassion is already inside you. It is a divine quality that becomes distorted only when the food police take the microphone. When you reconnect with that inner compassion, you reconnect with the part of you that reflects the image of God, the Universe, or whatever name you give to the sacred. Say those same gentle words to yourself with a mic drop.

From this place of gentleness, begin to identify your food rules. Consider writing them down in your journal. Then look at the statements your inner food police repeats: the criticisms, the warnings, the shaming messages. Most people feel an immediate discomfort and a spiritual dissonance because these messages are misaligned with love. That discomfort you feel is important. It is guidance. It is the quiet wisdom within you saying that there is a better way.

Finally, take each food police message and rewrite it into a compassionate affirmation. Let it be something that honors your body as a creation worthy of care. Let it sound like the voice of a loving guide. This is the work of liberation, the work of returning to the truth that your worth was never meant to be measured by rules, rigidity, or fear. This is deeply spiritual work, and it will continue to unfold gently within you each time you choose love over judgment.

Chapter Six

Discover the Satisfaction Factor and Savor the Good Gifts

"I can't get no..." *bum-bum-bum* "sat-is-faction." *bum-bum-bum.* Mick Jagger is singing about frustration for so many things in this Rolling Stones song—consumerism, sex, the pressures of society—but for me, it also captures the mood of diet culture. And now that the song is in both of our heads, let's chat about the importance of satisfaction in food.

My husband and I like to ask this question at dinner parties: "If it was your last day on Earth, what would you choose for your last meal?" Because we're food people, that last meal comes with an appetizer, entree, and dessert, and you're allowed to pair a beverage with each of these if you choose. You can choose anything you want. Here's the funny thing: I don't think we've ever said the same meal twice. Why? Because even if you have a favorite food, you may not always be in the mood for it. My mother makes the best lasagna in the world, but I probably don't want it for breakfast.

As I sit here right now, for my appetizer, I would choose the mozzarella sticks from The Spot in Galveston, Texas. They're basically the size of Twinkies, and one time I got the cheese to pull over two feet long! Delicious. I'd pair it with a tall Shiner beer served in a frozen glass. For my entree, I would choose my father-in-law's perfectly grilled veggie cheeseburgers with a side of my mother-in-law's cheesy broccoli and rice casserole, paired with a large glass of Montepulciano wine. And finally for dessert, my sister's famous key lime pie with a lovely hot cup of mint tea. Most of the time, I would choose my mother's aforementioned lasagna, and my sister, an award-winning pastry chef, almost always ends up being the creator of my dessert of choice. But right now, this would be the most satisfying meal.

Take a second to think about yours. What would be your last meal? Or maybe what is your favorite food? Is it something savory or something sweet? Is it a specific item from one of your favorite restaurants? Or is it a family recipe that's only made on special occasions? How does it feel to think about the food you love? How do you feel when you eat that food?

When I choose to eat something special, I allow myself to fully attend that moment because it simply feels so good to do so. It is the equivalent of being bear hugged by someone you've missed terribly or receiving kisses from a soft squishy puppy or getting into fresh clean sheets or putting in the final piece of the jigsaw puzzle or having the cat who ignores everyone else at the party jump in your lap. It feels good. It is blissful. It is one of life's little moments that gives us an instant dopamine hit and fills us with joy, and joy is an important part of satisfaction.

Intuitive eating would expand on satisfaction as more than just being fed; it's also about being fulfilled. It is the place where we are nourished, yes, but also gratified. Satisfaction is when you can end your meal feeling grounded and at peace without any sense of guilt or feeling of deprivation. It's being able to say, "That was enough. I am content."

If you were to name a diet, truly any diet in the history of time, a defining side effect of that diet would be the absence of satisfaction. Diets always require you to abstain from at least one thing (often many), which results in obsession, deprivation, and cravings. Satisfying those cravings is often looked at as "cheating" and a moral failure on the part of the dieter. Intuitive eating says not only should you *not* feel guilty about satisfaction, you should also *seek* it.

Forced Denial, Thy Name Is Diet Culture (Again)

There are many different reasons why we enjoy and choose the foods we do, and all of them are valid. Yet, we give less validity to satisfaction. In fact, we often actively work against allowing ourselves to be satisfied. Many of us feel, at best, over-indulgent, and at worst, guilty, simply for enjoying the pleasure of eating our favorite foods. This is heartbreaking.

How did we get to a place where satisfaction is seen as a bad thing? Why do we describe deliberate avoidance of satisfaction as strength or willpower? So much of this goes back to Chapter 2 and diet culture. In order for weight loss products to make a profit, they need their customers to believe the marketing campaigns that promise to "shed the pounds" if only you can avoid whatever food(s) that particular product is demonizing. If you are able to abstain, you're doing it right. If you are not able to abstain and instead attempt to satisfy your physical and emotional needs, you're doing it wrong. This is how every weight-loss product ensures that you are to blame instead of the snake oil they are selling because when you fail, it will be because you didn't try hard enough.

It is one of the more clever lies behind diet culture and one of the more heartbreaking ones because it is robbing us of our joy. Life is hard. Sometimes really, really hard. These weight-loss products, weight-loss influencers, and endless diets make it even harder. If we look closely, there are so many pleasurable things in life, but not many of them are actually required for our survival. Food is. We have the potential to live every day of our lives ensuring that our bodies survive by supplying it with food AND by achieving pleasure and satisfaction at the same time. It's a beautiful gift! We owe it to ourselves to fully embrace that gift and no longer tolerate or listen to the marketing campaigns that do not care about our quality of life.

As a therapist I'm curious by nature. It's part of my job and my training. I'm always curious about what's behind the statement of "I can't have that" or "I'm not a __ person." For example, when describing a particular dessert, I might hear "I'm not an ice cream person" or "I'm not a chocolate person." Maybe even "I'm not a someone-who-loves-dessert person." I realize that for some people, this may be true. However, I often suspect that these statements are more likely coming from a place of unworthiness and diet culture misinformation. That person doesn't believe they should get to have dessert because they didn't go to the gym, they shouldn't eat X number of calories, they haven't "earned" it, or something similar. (We'll talk about ingredient demonizing in Chapter 11.) Personally, I don't crave desserts or sweets the way I did when I tried to avoid them, but when I'm in the mood, I wholeheartedly enjoy dessert.

What about you? What about warm, fresh-out-of-the-oven chocolate chip cookies? Or crisp cannolis with fresh chocolate chip ricotta filling? Or how about apple cinnamon cobbler with a salty, buttery crust? When was the last time you had *real* ice cream? Try to be in a bad mood while eating ice cream. I double-scoop dare you.

Today I had a dark chocolate sea salt caramel truffle, and it was delightful. Heaven in a bite. Yet, it seems that the more decadent a dessert is, the more some may feel that it's sinful to eat it. Did I steal the truffle? No, of course not. So where is the sin? Where is the rationale for such guilt? Decadent foods, such as desserts, can and should have a place in our lives. We need to let go of the idea that we are being bad when we choose these foods because "being bad" is another example of food-police language derived from diet culture. I can tell you with confidence that ruining the pleasure of eating one of my sister's made-from-scratch, light, airy, piping hot, powdered sugar beignets by adding a side of guilt is the actual sin. The only thing that belongs on the side of those perfect little French donuts is chocolate sauce.

The Divine Gift of Satisfaction

As we've covered, satisfaction can mean many different things, and there are many factors to consider when deciding what to eat. It might be energy needs, medical dietary requirements or allergies, personal beliefs, accessibility, and more.

As a distance runner, satisfaction is meeting my energy needs before a long run or race. I have consistently had a big ol' bowl of pasta the night before a long run or race. The morning of the race, my go-to is peanut butter toast. This is because one, I know it will sustain me and fuel my body for endurance running, and two, runners know how quickly a run can turn real bad real quick if you've eaten the wrong thing… and you never want to be desperate for a bathroom miles from your destination. No bueno.

Satisfaction can be you realizing you haven't had many vegetables throughout the day, so before your evening main course, you have a lovely side salad with crisp lettuce and fresh veggies.

If you have Celiac disease and are unable to eat gluten or are vegan and choose not to have any animal products, then you will choose the food that is available and meets your dietary restrictions.

If you are not the primary cook in your home, then you will be eating (gratefully, I hope) whatever is cooked for you. Or maybe you're restricted to what's available in your local store or what your budget can support.

I don't meal prep. I understand why someone would meal

prep, and it sounds like a great time-saver, but I have severe food FOMO. Leftovers in our house will be eaten once but certainly not multiple times throughout the week. There are just too many foods to try. There is no way for me to know today what I will be in the mood for at the end of the week. Allowing myself to follow and satisfy my hunger matters to me. You can call it one of my guiding food values like we talked about in the last chapter. It's also why this intuitive eating principle is so important.

Satisfaction comes not only from the pleasure of taste and texture; it's also in finding that sweet spot between being hungry and being full. Providing yourself with ample portions of a balanced meal with proteins, carbs, fruits, veggies, and fats is likely going to give you that. Some foods are for my body. Some foods are for my soul. And I derive equal satisfaction from both.

Have you ever made something you were excited to share with someone? Did you watch them taste the first bite? Did you wait for their reaction and even if they gave you a positive one, did you solicit for even more positive feedback? **There is something beautiful about feeding others. It's giving a piece of ourselves to another. It's sharing a part of who we are, and we delight when someone takes pleasure from that.** There is satisfaction in the altruism and hospitality of sharing love and generosity.

In the Jewish tradition, there is *Oneg Shabbat,* or "Sabbath Delight," which is a social gathering typically held on Friday or Saturday evenings to celebrate the Sabbath with fellowship and a communal meal. A rabbi described it to me as a time to pause. "There's a sweetness in that pause, and in that sweetness, we serve food to each other and enjoy food together."

She went on to share a beautiful example of how food itself holds so much power. She said, "When I am kneading the dough to make challah bread, I let go of all the stress from the week. I'll also make the bread with my children and think about how the experience of life's sweet moments are all woven into this beautiful bread." She went on to say, "It's our God-given sacred responsibility to give ourselves that nourishment, and it's counter-culture to deny ourselves." There is pleasure, satisfaction, meaning, and purpose throughout the experience.

There are many faith traditions that acknowledge satisfaction in eating. In Sikhism, food is understood as a gift so the soul can live, serve, and connect more fully to the divine. Enjoyment of food is not considered sinful or indulgent. Instead, it is meant to be received with gratitude, humility, and balance. One of the most defining features of the *gurdwara,* or the Sikh religious building or place of worship, is a large communal meal called the *langar*. The *langar* is a free meal offered to visitors regardless of religious background. Everyone sits together on the floor and enjoys simple, nourishing, and satisfying foods. Warm bread, lentils, vegetables, and sweets are meant to be enjoyed, not rushed or moralized. Satisfaction here is not just physical but spiritual and communal. Eating until you are comfortably full is expected and encouraged because the meal is meant to sustain and honor the body.

Within Indigenous and earth-based traditions, members of the culture often treat food as a sacred relationship. Satisfaction is not only allowed but honored because the act of eating connects people to the land, their ancestors, the seasons, and their community. Pleasure is woven into gratitude rituals, storytelling, and feasting. Food is meant to be enjoyed as part of belonging to the web of life. In this way, intuitive eating's invitation to discover the satisfaction factor is not a modern rebellion but a return to ancient wisdom that understands nourishment as sensory, relational, and sacred.

Returning to a Life of Satisfaction

I'm not sure about reincarnation. I think it's a cool idea, and I wouldn't mind coming back and trying again as a (hopefully) more enlightened version of myself. But if it isn't the case, then this is all we get. Even if we are reincarnated, the *you* right now is the only version of you who will have the chance to enjoy the specific foods in your life. Right now. No other you will be able to eat that special once-a-year family recipe that's been passed down for generations. **This one chance at making our lives meaningful and joyful is exactly that—one chance.** Denying yourself your favorite foods because of diet culture rules about "good" and "bad" food robs you of the satisfaction of *now,* and eating only kale will not allow you to live forever. None of us are getting out of this life alive. YOLO, friends. YOLO.

Whether it's diet culture or some other reason (most likely derived from diet culture), too many of us have forgotten how to be satisfied or how to allow ourselves to be satisfied from our food choices. But like any skill, you can reconnect with your satisfaction factor, and the co-founders of intuitive eating have created five steps to regain that pleasure of eating.

Step 1: Ask yourself what you really want.

This is harder than it sounds because most of us have had so many rules in our minds about what we "should" want that checking in about our actual taste preferences seems foreign. Oftentimes we settle for the diet dessert and tell ourselves it's sufficient, but it's never going to be as good as the real thing. It is rarely going to completely satisfy the craving. (This is why I take issue with the concept of substitutions. Thanks again, diet culture.)

This will be an unpopular opinion, but if what you really want is a pizza, then putting a tablespoon of marinara on a rice cake isn't gonna cut it. Any time you choose something that says "light" or "low fat" or "guilt free," it is robbing you of the satisfaction factor *if you don't like it as much.* If you sincerely do prefer those versions, then go for it. But it's likely you prefer the real deal and you're choosing those other versions because you think you should. When we choose the substitute out of guilt, we usually end up eating more than we intended and feel uncomfortable, we don't feel satisfied, and we still crave the real-deal version we originally wanted.

Do you remember the SnackWells desserts that came out during the low-fat craze of the 1990s? These were objectively terrible. Just about everyone would agree that these would never be preferred over real cookies and cakes. Even still, their most popular product was their Devil's food cookie cakes, which I once heard described as "eating a chocolate cupcake whose soul had been sucked out." However, at that time, a low-fat diet was all the rage, and people sold the idea that SnackWells was a healthy substitute for chocolate cravings. As a result, their line of low-fat snacks, including the signature Devil's food cookie cake, blew up to nearly $500 million in 1995, money earned because we collectively decided to settle for substitutions instead of real satisfaction. But SnackWells would not endure. Over the decades, low-fat fell out of fashion, and the brand was discontinued in 2022. This isn't to say that there aren't new substitutes in its place, but I hope it's due in part to people learning to give themselves what they truly want.

Step 2: Discover the pleasure of the palate.

I love this step. Through the years, I've seen this step be mind-blowing for patients when they actually stop and think about the experience of eating and truly savoring food.

Intuitive eating encourages the intentional act of slowing down without distraction and deliberately tuning in to the sensations of the eating experience. In the current day and age, this isn't an easy ask. We're too caught up in our to-do lists, not to mention the super computer we carry around with us at all times, to focus on one activity at a time, let alone if that activity is eating. But **allowing pleasure to be a legitimate part of our nourishment can be a life-changing way of shifting our experience with eating.**

This is done through taste, texture, aroma, appearance, temperature, and volume or filling capacity.

- ***Taste.*** When we think of taste, we may ask ourselves, is the taste enjoyable or unpleasant? Is it sweet or sour or salty? It's always fascinating to learn what people crave, and interestingly, most are in the sweet or the salty camp. Many people might make the mistake of assuming that this is really all that matters when it comes to satisfaction, but many find that these next aspects are equally, if not even more, important.

- ***Texture.*** Texture may be the most unique preference of all. Think about how many times you've heard (or maybe even experienced for yourself) that the texture of a food is so off-putting that it makes it unpalatable. For me, that's oatmeal. Can't do it. It always smells delightful, but I can't get past the texture.

- ***Aroma.*** Smells can sometimes make or break even the willingness to try a food. And yet, if the aroma is pleasant, it can instantaneously create a desire for that food. Think of freshly baked cookies coming out of the oven or popcorn at the movie theatre.

- ***Appearance.*** As chefs, my sister and brother-in-law will tell you that appearance is everything. The presentation of the food delivered to the table matters. It indicates the care and effort that was put into the preparation, and expert chefs take great pains to make their plates creative and beautiful. Have you ever chosen your menu item at a restaurant after seeing a plate being delivered to a nearby table? Why would you do this? You have no idea how it tastes yet, but the appearance of it was appealing to you and therefore likely to enhance your satisfaction with the meal.

- ***Temperature.*** Many of us find that the temperature of the meal may matter and influence our satisfaction based on our own temperatures. It's less likely that you will want hot soup while sitting on a patio in the summer in Texas, for example.
- ***Volume.*** The volume or filling capacity of a meal encourages us to practice honoring our hunger and check in with how much we need to feel satisfied. If it's been several hours since your last meal, then a handful of nuts likely won't be enough to satisfy you. On the other hand, if you've just finished a balanced dinner, you may only desire two cookies for dessert instead of four to feel satisfied.

Step 3: Make your eating experience more enjoyable.

This step encourages eating while we are not distracted so we can experience the satisfaction that food provides. Ideally, this involves a pleasant environment, taking our time, savoring, checking in with our hunger and fullness cues, and having a variety of foods.

One way I achieve this is to eat in an area that's free of clutter. I once heard the expression "messy space, messy mind," so I like to take a couple extra minutes to clear and wipe down the space before settling in to enjoy the meal. For example, I happen to make very good pasta. I have a variety of recipes I've perfected, and I'm always experimenting with new ones. Whenever I'm particularly proud of a pasta dish I've prepared, I make sure to serve it in these gorgeous ceramic bowls I found in Positano, Italy. They're handpainted with bright yellow lemons and blue detailing. When my dining space is clear, I can focus on the amazing food I lovingly prepared and enjoy the art of the dish holding my meal. It all makes the experience extra special and makes me feel fancy. This is an infinitely better experience than doom scrolling while trying to have a nice meal.

Step 4: Don't settle.

If you don't like something, don't eat it. (See Step 1 about substitutions.) I want to like mushrooms. They're often served in salad recipes at some of my favorite salad places, and they're nearly always on a veggie pizza. As a vegetarian, I feel it's my responsibility to embrace all vegetables, but I genuinely don't care for them. (And yes, I know mushrooms are technically a fungi, but they are widely considered a vegetable in culinary and nutritional context.) So when I order my veggie omelet, I just say, "No mushrooms, please," and we all move on with our lives.

Step 5: Does it still taste good?

This step advises that you check-in throughout the eating experience. It's possible the first bites of something are really pleasurable because maybe you're super hungry or maybe you've been craving that particular food. But as you continue to eat, is it still good? Is it meeting the taste, texture, aroma, appearance, and temperature qualities that are satisfying at this moment? If not, repeat Step 4 and don't settle.

* * * *

When a new brewery opened up in our area, my husband and I went to check it out. We grabbed a couple of beers at the bar and found a seat at one of the long community tables. The brewery had an industrial, large, open-concept design with lots of natural light and high ceilings. The bar itself was on one side of the space, and a stage for live music filled the other side. It was new, clean, and busy with families with kiddos and doggos at nearly every table.

Beyond food and drinks, they also had a board game section. We played several of the games, including a round of Guess Who, and completed two puzzles. As we sat there enjoying our beer and pizza and playing a game, it occurred to me that we could be doing exactly the same thing at home for a lot less money. So why weren't we? Why do so many of us like going to restaurants? There are hundreds of thousands of them across the US, so there must be a reason. We could always go to the grocery store and make all of our meals at home, so what does going out to eat provide for us that eating at home does not? I would argue that, yes, it's the food, but it's also so much more than that; it's the satisfaction derived from the *experience* of eating.

The environment you are in and the people you are with adds to the satisfaction of the eating experience. Restaurants create space for conversations, celebrations, and togetherness. The atmosphere, flavors, and service make the experience feel special and offer relief from daily responsibilities. From street tacos to sushi, dining out also opens the door to different cultures, traditions, and creativity through food. Many people are drawn to the ritual and rhythm of going out. Think about everything you notice, such as the music, the lighting, and the decor. It's all part of the experience, and it all has the power to enhance our satisfaction.

I love to go out to eat. I love trying new restaurants. I even have an Instagram page and a website where I document my experiences. This isn't about any real desire to have people read them; it's just always been fun for me. My very first job was as a waitress at my friend's family restaurant. I was only fifteen years old, and the experience of working there really nurtured my love of restaurants and eating out. It was a 1950s themed restaurant with big red booths and a black-and-white checkered floor that specialized in burgers and milkshakes. The restaurant even had an Elvis impersonator on Friday nights.

Since this first job, I've worked in many restaurants and bars over the years, including fine dining restaurants where the rules of conduct and presentation for servers were beyond strict; they were militant. I've scooped ice cream, slung drinks, and pulled pints. I learned how to make the perfect espresso and cappuccino. I have a million memories from all of these jobs, and at the heart of all of them, it's about fellowship, breaking bread, serving others, and just enjoying what it means to be alive. It's about the satisfaction of life.

The element of mindfulness is integral to satisfaction in these environments. When we go out to eat, we are pausing our to-do list. We have scheduled this protected time to eat in companionship with others and be present in the moment. We are attuned to our senses and focused on what's placed on our table and the people sitting around it. This is also one space where we often allow ourselves to be satisfied. Because make no mistake—this is a spiritual moment. **When we are fully present and attentive and have given ourselves permission to engage fully in the current moment, we are cultivating a mindfulness practice.**

Mindfulness is found in many faiths and cultures around the world. The spiritual practice of mindfulness can improve both mental and physical health, deepen our sense of presence and wakefulness, foster gratitude, encourage self-acceptance, and cultivate a sense of unity, belonging, and connectedness. True satisfaction and nourishment affect more than the body; they touch the mind, heart, and spirit.

Practice Discovering the Satisfaction Factor

When was the last time you truly enjoyed a meal? What would it be like if you were able to slow down enough to fully taste your food and allow joy and ease to settle into your body? What might come up in that moment both emotionally and spiritually? Consider what might open up in your life if you believed that satisfaction was not indulgent but part of the Universe's compassionate design for you. Imagine the freedom that comes with trusting that your body was created to receive pleasure, and let it be a reminder that you are meant to experience goodness, not just endure survival. Take a moment to journal on the thoughts that come up.

This may feel like very unfamiliar territory. That's okay. Diet culture has taught many of us to treat pleasure with suspicion and to see satisfaction as something to resist, or worse, something you need to earn. Without any judgment, begin noticing where those rules show up in your daily eating. You might take a moment to list five foods you have been forcing yourself to eat out of guilt or ideas about what you "should" choose. Then pick one and allow yourself to skip the substitution and fully enjoy the version your body genuinely prefers.

You can also practice a mindful tasting exercise to help reconnect you with the sacred nature of eating. Slow down the pace of your next meal and allow yourself to experience texture, aroma, and flavor with full attention. Notice the way your body responds when you remove judgment and make room for gratitude. This kind of presence is a spiritual discipline. It teaches you to meet your body with reverence and reminds you that satisfaction is not the enemy of health but a pathway toward wholeness and joy.

Finally, you know that restaurant you've been wondering about? Perhaps the one you see on your drive home from work or the one that popped up in your social media feed? It's time. Go and practice the five steps to regain the pleasure of eating discussed in this chapter. And if the server asks if you are celebrating anything, you can enthusiastically say, "Yes, I'm celebrating a little milestone in learning to savor life, starting with tonight's dinner."

Chapter Seven

Feel Your Fullness and Listen to Your Body's Inner Wisdom

I was running an eating disorder clinic in Dallas the first time I heard the term *interoceptive awareness*. We were launching a new therapeutic model, one we'd adapted from an existing model called the Unified Protocol. Our model was going to be used with eating disorders, and it included a component of interoceptive exposure to help increase someone's interoceptive awareness.

Interoceptive awareness is your ability to sense and understand the internal signals of your body. *Interoception* comes from the Latin root *intero-* ("inside") and *-ception* ("to sense or perceive"). So interoception literally means sensing what's inside. It refers to your ability to feel internal body sensations like your heartbeat, breathing, and hunger. Think of it as your brain's internal listening system that helps you notice bodily cues. Interoception also includes noticing nervous system responses connected to safety and stress, such as butterflies in the stomach, a racing heart, sweaty palms, tightness in the chest, or even numbness and shutdown. These sensations are always happening in the background, and interoceptive awareness is what allows you to tune into them and respond in a way that supports both your body and your sense of safety. It's pretty cool, right? You can imagine just how excited we were to bring interoceptivity into eating disorder treatment. We felt it could help a lot of people.

As the director of the clinic, it was primarily my responsibility to oversee the administrative and operational functions of the clinic. However, every now and again, perhaps if we were short-staffed, I would find myself running a group therapy session. Now, I love running groups. I think group therapy is wildly underrated in mainstream culture. I also (humbly) happen to be very good at it. However, if I found myself needing to facilitate a group interoceptive exposure exercise, I was less than enthusiastic.

As a therapist, I think interoceptive awareness is incredibly powerful, informative, and constructive. But as a therapist leading the group, it's not easy. One of the tenets of any kind of exposure therapy is that the therapist is there with you throughout the experience. Not only are you, the therapist, present with the patient, you are also participating with them. Whatever discomfort I asked the patients to put themselves through, I needed to also do myself.

I get it. It is important. But I don't always like it.

One of the interoceptive exercises that stands out to me is the breathing-through-the-straw exercise. The exercise is designed to stimulate the sensation of shortness of breath. Recreating this sensation can often trigger anxiety or panic along with physical symptoms: air hunger, chest tightness, and/or dizziness. All of these are unpleasant to experience, but the benefits are worth it. When we expose ourselves to the discomfort in this safe environment under the guidance of a trained clinician, we learn that while these sensations are uncomfortable, they're not dangerous. This results in a reduction of the fear around these symptoms and an increased tolerance for them. Even though I wouldn't be the first to volunteer to repeat this exercise, it teaches invaluable information about how to increase awareness of our internal sensations and learn from them.

The primary objective of this principle is to "feel your fullness," which is all about noticing the subtle bodily signals that tell you when you're comfortably satisfied. In other words, it's about improving interoceptive awareness. If you review the principles we've already discussed, many of them are specifically geared towards increasing interoceptive awareness. You've been slowly working on this skill in Chapter 3 with honoring your hunger; Chapter 6 in discovering the satisfaction factor; this chapter on feeling your fullness, and soon in Chapter 10 with movement and finding harmony and flow of your body, mind, and spirit..

Many people have learned to disconnect from their body's signals due to chronic dieting and/or diet culture's messaging around trying to control our bodies versus listening to them. If you've learned to power through meals without checking in, then your ability to feel and respond to gentle fullness cues are most likely blunted. This is why the founders of intuitive eating created so many opportunities for people to reconnect with their bodies over and over again; interoceptive awareness is critical to learning to trust the divine wisdom inherent in the body.

A key point in honoring your hunger is that our biology and God's design signal to us when we are hungry so that we nourish ourselves to sustain our bodies' needs. The same is true for *feeling your fullness.* When we can tune in to the way our body feels and be present, patient, and trusting in God's miraculous design that is the human body, we can trust when to eat and when to stop.

Trusting Your Gut

I need to confess something: I have not perfected the intuitive eating principles in my own life. Now don't get me wrong—I live them and teach them daily. But I'm not at 100 percent; I'm going to put myself at 97.5% percent. While some people may attain 100 percent, it feels unattainable to me. I was deeply immersed in diet culture for a long time. Even when you know all the research and all the scams and all the clinical best practices, old habits die hard. The principle of "feel your fullness" still throws me a curve ball from time to time. But this is about progress and not perfection on your journey back to self.

What still gets me every now and then is being a lifelong member of the "Clean Your Plate" Club. Pretty much everyone in my generation is a member of this club, but it's certainly not exclusive to my generation. We grew up knowing that you cleaned your plate because not doing so was wasteful and a sign of ingratitude to whomever prepared the meal. So in order to stuff that last bite of meatloaf down, we collectively learned to ignore how full we felt and just keep going lest we seem ungrateful for Grandma's efforts.

Fortunately, over time, I learned how to stop and check in with how I'm feeling during the eating experience. I can now sense when I'm nearing satisfaction and then stop eating before I get too full. But membership in the "Clean Your Plate" Club has no expiration date, and one particular night, I found myself eating more takeout pizza than I wanted or needed.

Now there's a reason pizza is such a fan favorite for so many people: Even the pickiest eaters usually like a slice of plain cheese pizza, even though there's nothing plain about it. The combination of a robust marinara with flavors of garlic, basil, and oregano topped with melty, stretchy mozzarella resting on a buttery crusty bread is really hard to top. Having been to the birthplace of pizza in Naples, Italy, as well as growing up in New Jersey and going to school in New York, I know my pizza. I no longer live in the northeast, and although I don't miss the cold climate, I lament the loss of an endless supply of solid pizza joints on every corner. Here in Texas, it's much harder to find, but we've come across a few reliable local options.

On the night in question, we ordered a NY style cheesy pie, extra large, and brought it home to enjoy with family. Pizza always smells amazing, and this was no exception. Opening the warm box and getting the first whiff of the savory aroma definitely had me eager for that first slice. It was piping hot, and the cheese weighed the slice down so much it required two hands to eat it. That's just the best. It was tasty, had a good amount of mozzarella, a chewy crust with some browned edges, and a decent marinara, not too sweet and not too salty.

When I'd finished my first slice, I wanted a second. About half way through the second slice, I silently and gently completed the taste check and satiety check that Tribole and Reysch recommend.

Did it taste as good? *No.* It had smelled really good when I opened the box, and I did really like the first slice, but I've definitely had much better pizza.

Was I still hungry? *No.* I was already full. And while there are plenty of food items I have zero problem saving for later (half a sandwich, leftover pasta, and so on), putting back a half eaten piece of pizza just doesn't seem right. Because the "Clean Your Plate" Club voice in my mind shouted at me not to throw it away, I finished it and was subsequently uncomfortably full.

Why would I share this with you? I'm an expert in this area, and I want you to trust me and all of the other brilliant clinicians doing this work. So why would I share that I'm not perfect at this? Because the majority of us will have experiences like this even if, like me, we've been doing this for over a decade.

You can learn the skills and be really, really good at them. They can change your life. I sincerely mean that with all my heart. But even with your learned skills, you can still have an experience where you aren't as perfectly in tune as you hoped, and that is completely okay. We're human after all.

Further, feeling your fullness is tough. It's asking you to trust your body and listen to what it's saying. It's not lost on me that "trust yourself" is a difficult concept for some (see the pizza story above). I've also had patients clearly state the emphatic opposite: "I can't trust myself" or "I don't trust myself." There are so many reasons why we get to this point. A likely culprit is the diet culture that forced false messages upon us and taught us to ignore our inner wisdom. Another may have been the external food police in your family or community, that voice at our own tables growing up: "You don't need that" or "You've already had enough." Certainly both of these are likely suspects as to how we may come to lose self-trust. If we believe there is something bigger than us in this Universe, we are trusting something beyond proof. That is the same posture intuitive eating asks of us when we stop outsourcing trust to external rules and begin listening inward. It may be confusing, but it's also beautiful.

Returning to the Wisdom of the Body

One of my colleagues and I recently had a fascinating conversation on this topic during lunch. She is a Muslim woman and a follower of the Islamic faith. She shared with me that in their tradition, Muslims view eating as very simple: You eat to fuel your body, and you eat enough to get full. Food is eaten in order to prevent hunger and ensure the body remains healthy. The way they do this is with the one-third rule: one-third of the stomach for food, one-third for water or drink, and one-third left empty for air (breathing/space). The purpose behind the rule is a spiritual discipline that encourages mindfulness, gratitude, and self-control, as well as preventing physical discomfort that could distract from the spiritual discipline. Excessive amounts of food are discouraged because it would create discomfort and interfere with spiritual connectedness.

She elaborated on this point, stating that doing anything to hurt the body could be perceived as a sin. This would include overeating, yes, but undereating or overexercising would also be seen as equally harmful and not liked in the eyes of God. "Mohammed told of moderation in all things," she said, "in your job, in your relationships, and in eating habits. When you're in better health, it allows you to go after spiritual pursuits. Food can still be pleasurable, like right now as we sit here and enjoy two big pieces of pie, but excessive indulgence hurts the body. We take care of our body because God entrusted us with this body." This ties together the last chapter about satisfaction and our current discussion about feeling fullness. The moment our needs are satisfied often aligns with the moment our bodies' needs are fulfilled.

In order to feel your fullness, you have to work on building and enhancing self-trust. All of the principles we've discussed thus far are steps on that journey, and it's not necessarily linear. It can certainly go backwards and forwards a few times along the way. I know I have. As Bob Goff states in *Undistracted,* "We're following a God we can't see, for a lifetime we can't measure, to a heaven we can't comprehend… is it any wonder we're all a little muddled?" Yet, a fundamental connection that can make self-trust easier is remembering where we came from. I don't mean your city of birth, although if that helps, then by all means. What I mean is remembering that you are a child of the Universe and to take care of yourself as such.

I hope you noticed the poem at the start of this book. I stumbled upon a quote from this poem by Max Ehrmann on a magnet while I was standing in line at the grocery store over twenty years ago: "Be gentle with yourself. You are a child of the universe, no less than the trees and the stars. In the noisy confusion of life. Keep peace in your soul." It spoke to me in that moment, and after finding the full poem, the message continued to resonate with me deeply. The poem is titled "Desiderata," meaning "things to be desired." Max Ehrmann studied law at Harvard but preferred to write plays and poetry. In 1927, he wrote "Desiderata" as a gift to himself stemming from a desire to put into words his philosophical beliefs. I still find it the most grounding text I've ever read. It has realigned my perspective countless times when I found myself lost in the noisy confusion of life and reminds me that "no doubt the Universe is unfolding as it should." It centers me towards my values and greater purpose and helps me continue to honor my body and give it everything it needs to live that purpose.

At the heart of many spiritual teachings is the belief that we are created with purpose and inherent goodness. Rebuilding self-trust starts by acknowledging that your inner voice is not your enemy, and while it may be clouded, it's not broken. You were created with wisdom, intuition, and the ability to choose well.

When we all came into this world, we were born with the inherent knowledge of hunger and fullness. Babies are born with innate interoceptive awareness and will communicate, loudly, when they are hungry and will then communicate when they're done. This seems to be pretty stark evidence that God had a pretty solid design.

Rebuilding self-trust means treating your body not as a project, but as a partner. **In a spiritual sense, trusting yourself is an act of returning to the divine truth that you are enough and always have been.** After rejecting a diet culture that has told you otherwise, rebuilding self-trust may feel unfamiliar at first. Perhaps an initial thought to get you started is as simple as: "This food feels nourishing today, and I feel satisfied," or "I feel drawn to joy, not restriction." Instead of seeing the body as something to be controlled or corrected, see it as an instrument of spiritual experience.

It's important to remember that feeling your fullness is very nuanced. It isn't as black-and-white as it may sound. "Am I full or not?" is way too oversimplified. It's by intentionally slowing down and increasing your attunement to your body, both your physical and emotional sensations, that you can develop a better sense of the patterns of your body and how it feels. From there you can determine if those sensations are pleasant or unpleasant. Your experience with this will take practice, so creating an environment where that's easier is especially helpful in the early stages of this approach. Revisit Chapter 6 for additional suggestions on this particular topic. Most importantly, though, turn your attention inward and remember to do so with patience and without judgment or expectations.

I mention the word "expectations" here because diet culture spends a lot of its time telling us we need less food than we actually do. When we start to tune in to our bodies and be guided by our fullness sensations, we may be surprised by how much or how little we eat at any given time. For example, I have had several experiences where I have felt ravenous. After I've started eating, I hit a fullness level where I no longer need any more to feel satisfied and end up eating less than I thought I might. And that's okay. Then of course, the converse of that has occurred where I didn't think I was that hungry but after eliminating distractions and staying attuned, I realized I was much hungrier than I thought. So I allowed myself to eat more than I initially thought I would. That's okay, too. In both instances, I am listening and paying attention to my body's needs, which differ based on any number of things.

There is a beautiful philosophy within many Indigenous and Earth-based spiritual traditions that believes the body is an extension of the Earth. In other words, the same elements that flow through the Earth also flow through our bodies. Therefore, listening intuitively to our bodies and paying attention to our hunger and fullness cues can be compared to listening to the rhythms of nature itself.

In these traditions, eating is so much more than eating only for biological survival. It's part of the give-and-take relationship of nature. "Take only what you need, and use all that you take" is a common teaching across many Native traditions. This is in line with their values of balance and reciprocity with the gifts the Earth and nature provide.

What a gorgeous way of looking at ourselves! Our bodies are part of the Earth, and therefore, just as nature communicates through rhythm and flow, our bodies speak through hunger and fullness *when we learn how to listen.* By embracing this philosophy, you can anticipate a shift that takes place in your sense of security, worthiness, and overall sense of self.

Practice Feeling Your Fullness

This chapter is all about listening inward. This principle invites you to listen inward with gentleness and curiosity. Your body is always communicating with you and invites you to begin increasing your interoceptive awareness and begin to notice the internal shifts that happen as you approach satisfaction. Perhaps your pace slows or you begin to notice all of the flavors of your food. Tune into sensations in your stomach. Has your heart rate increased or slowed? Ask yourself what your body is telling you. When you begin to observe how your body speaks to you in these moments, you may feel a sense of gratitude rise. It's pretty cool when we give our bodies the attention they deserve.

It's important to remember that checking your fullness is not a test of willpower. This pause is not about stopping early or eating less; it's about building the relationship between you and your body. If you are willing to pause and listen to your body's needs, you will find there's an inner knowing we're created with. When you listen closely, your fullness cues become a conversation between your body and your spirit and a reminder that you were made with intention and care.

Consider writing about what fullness feels like for you. Describe it as information, not as something that should make you feel proud or ashamed. This step transforms fullness into a spiritual dialogue as you look inward. It invites you to trust the body you were given and the wisdom placed within you.

As you practice tuning in to these subtle cues, you will discover that your fullness is not the end of a meal. It is a moment of alignment. It is the point where nourishment, presence, and trust meet. And it is here, in this tender space, that you begin to remember that your body and spirit are always working together to guide you toward wholeness.

Chapter Eight

Cope with Your Emotions with Kindness and Nurture Your Spirit

Emotional eating has gotten a bad rap. Yes, I am taking a strong position that it is not the crisis you have been led to believe it is. Let me explain.

Someone you care about is grieving the loss of someone they love. As is tradition in many cultures, it is common for mourners to bring trays of food to the home of the bereaved. We do this out of a desire to help and out of concern for their wellbeing as they grieve. But mostly, we do this out of love.

When you're deciding on what type of casserole to bring, you're not concerned about emotional eating. You're about to attend a memorial, and therefore, people will be highly emotional. And what will you say after you share your condolences? I suspect it will be something like, "Can I fix you a plate?" Further, when you fix that plate, you won't intentionally skip over the higher calorie offerings in favor of crudité with low-fat dressing. No, you'll look specifically for your friend's favorite foods and pile the plate high with the food that feels like a hug when you eat it.

Don't get me wrong, I love raw carrots. But **when someone is in the depths of sadness, I'm not going to hand them a cold, hard carrot. I'm going to hand them a warm, soft cookie.**

Now imagine you are the bereaved. Someone who cares about you just fixed you a plate of some comfort food (comfort is in the name for a reason), say a large serving of homemade baked macaroni and cheese. You agree to the offer because even though you have less of an appetite, you know you need to eat, and it is usually one of your favorites.

While you are eating this, Aunt Susan walks over and says, "Be careful, honey, there's a ton of fat and calories in that dish. You don't want to have to cope with gaining weight on top of everything else you're going through."

Are you horrified? I hope so. The food police have no place here, and yet, how many times have you been made to feel bad about coping with food? How many times have you made yourself feel bad about coping with food?

Consider these other scenarios.

You have a terrible day at work and get home late so you order yourself and your family a hot, cheesy pizza. Or you break up with your significant other, so your sibling comes over with some freshly baked brownies to cheer you up. Or you didn't get the promotion you were promised, so your friends take you out for chips, salsa, and margaritas.

Yes, emotional eating can be problematic when it is the *only* tool in the toolkit. Can you imagine if massages were the only way to ease your anxiety? Unless you are very wealthy and travel with a masseuse, I don't know how feasible this would be. Same with food. No one is saying every time you feel stressed, you should only and always cope with it with chips, salsa, and margaritas. But you also can't convince me it is in anyone's best interest to add feeling like crap about yourself because you ate something a bit more indulgent than usual to get yourself through a hard day.

Enter the next principle: cope with your emotions with kindness and nurture your spirit. To effectively move through the hard times, we need both parts. We need to address the emotion in the moment and nurture our spirit along the way. When we do this, we have multiple tools at our disposal and can come out the other side of the emotion in a more loving, kinder, and stronger way.

Why the Hard Work Is Oftentimes the Most Important

One of the items in a therapist's toolkit is something called the Feelings Wheel. It's a circular, often brightly-colored visual tool that aims at assisting patients in identifying and articulating feelings. You'll find some variation of it in most therapists' offices as either a paper handout, wall poster, or even a throw pillow or an area rug. Why would this be so popular? Because it's harder than it sounds for many of us to name and articulate how we actually feel at any given moment. Think about it: When someone asks how you're doing, what is the most common answer? "Fine." Right? I suppose that's sufficient for the cashier at the grocery store, but it's lacking in substance for anyone who is genuinely interested in how you are doing. Therapists won't let you get away with "fine." The Feelings Wheel has all of the basic emotions (sad, happy, surprised, bad, fearful, angry, and disgusted) at the center, while the outer circles have much more nuanced adjectives, such as lonely, playful, critical, and rejected.

This tool isn't necessary only for children or adolescents. **Grown adults have difficulty putting into words how they actually feel because most of us are so busy in our day-to-day routine that we don't pause to think about our emotional state.** Additionally, very few of us received any kind of formal social-emotional instruction growing up. Even in the districts and states that offer social-emotional instruction as part of their educational curriculum, it's typically offered only at the early childhood and elementary levels. Meanwhile, we know our brains are not done developing until our mid-twenties, so that's a lot of missed opportunities to develop proficiency in identifying and communicating feelings. Combine this deficiency in articulating our feelings with the fact that life is really hard, and we can at times be flooded with multiple feelings at once. It's easy to see why it's essential to first identify the feeling or feelings and then cope with them in a safe and positive way.

The trouble is that at times, our emotions can be really intimidating. Frankly, it is sometimes just much easier to bury, suppress, and ignore difficult feelings than to address them. Some people are really well practiced at this. But friends, let me offer this to you, and it's backed by a therapist's guarantee: burying feelings will not work forever. It's like shoving everything into a junk drawer; even if you can ignore it, the mess is still there. The mess builds and builds, and it takes more and more effort to get the drawer to close until one day, you open the drawer and a rubber band, a battery, and a takeout menu attack you all at once.

Nurture Your Spirit, Expand Your Toolkit

Coping with food isn't terrible, but it can be harmful when it's your only go-to for when you are struggling. Additionally, if you find yourself eating frequently even when you're not biologically hungry, it is worth exploring what feelings are coming up. Or more likely, what feelings are you trying to keep down? Guilt and shame around food often leads us right back into the dieting-cycle hamster wheel. Complicating matters even further, research tells us that dieting is a predictor of emotional eating. When we diet, we don't trust our biological cues, so we inevitably end up eating more even if we're not biologically hungry because we're no longer in tune with said cues. This leads to feelings of guilt and shame, and we diet again. And round and round we go. In fact, a 2013 study published in *The American Journal of Clinical Nutrition* analyzed data from 35,641 adults (8,580 men and 27,061 women) and found that both former and current dieters exhibited higher emotional eating scores compared to individuals with no history of dieting. So let's spend a bit of time discussing and developing other methods to cope with our emotions. A great place to start is asking yourself what you have tried in the past that's been successful.

In her book *Big Magic,* best-selling author Elizabeth Gilbert says, "We all need an activity that is beyond the mundane and that takes us out of our established and limiting roles in society (mother, employee, neighbor, brother, boss, etc.)." She references the Gospel of Thomas and says, "If you bring forth what is within you, what you bring forth will save you. If you don't bring forth what is within you, what you don't bring forth will destroy you." There's a lot to unpack here.

All too often, we get caught up in the mundane and forget that our spirit needs our attention, too. Maybe as a kid you used to paint or craft, take dance class or play a team sport, read books or write your own stories, play an instrument or sing. But somewhere along the way, going to school or working or having children of your own took over all of your time and energy. So now you focus only on those mundane tasks, and there's nothing left for your spirit. That doesn't mean you're no longer interested in any of those activities or that your spirit doesn't need nurturing anymore; it means that you're neglecting at least one aspect of your spiritual hunger. Remember Chapter 3?

Without an outlet, emotionally difficult situations can more easily burden your spirit. Suddenly we find ourselves full of uncomfortable emotions, and we don't know what to do with them, how to express them, or how to work through them. So we eat to address our need to *do* something, and eating is all that we've allowed ourselves to do anymore. We're not bringing forth these emotions in a forward-moving way, so they're destroying us. We've limited our lives to such an extent that we have no life outside of the mundane.

When our spirit feels full and cared for, we can more easily

care for our emotional needs as they arise. That's why nurturing the spirit is so important.

As I mentioned before, I'm a runner. I feel a significant disturbance in my mood, anxiety, and sleep if I don't get a couple runs in during the week. So for me that's an essential coping skill, and it nurtures my spirit. However, I also love to constantly learn new things. In the last few years, I've taken drum lessons, creative writing classes, and Italian lessons. These give me a sense of joy and purpose so that when the hard times come, and of course they do, I have things to distract me and be a light on days when I feel like a black cloud is stalking me.

Think about the things that bring you joy and peace, that make your life feel full and your spirit sated. Sometimes food for pleasure and comfort is the right choice. Other times the right choice is movement, deep breathing, yoga, gardening, reading, watching a funny movie or video, cuddling your pets, coloring or drawing, prayer or spending time with loved ones, or anything else you've found that works for you.

Understanding the right way to nurture your spirit can be tough, especially if you've cut yourself off from joy and peace for a long time. Maybe you're feeling a bit stuck or unsure about what these interests or activities could be for you. Elizabeth Gilbert addresses this as well:

> ...but surely something wonderful is sheltered inside you. I say this with all confidence because I happen to believe we are all walking repositories of buried treasure... The Universe buries strange jewels within us all, and then stands back to see if we can find them. The hunt to uncover those jewels—that's creative living.

Creativity is about engaging the imagination, expressing your inner world, and making meaning. Science now confirms what many spiritual and cultural traditions have long taught, which is that doing something creative is a healing act. As you think about what activities to re-engage with, consider adding at least one creative outlet for your spirit.

What if you just really don't like doing many things and never have? How can you still nurture your spirit and have an emotional outlet? Consider the best way to prepare eggs. When people ask Gretchen Rubin, author of *The Happiness Project,* about the best path towards happiness, she responds: "What is the best way to cook an egg?" Her humorous point is well made in that everyone likes their eggs made a different way, just as each of our paths toward happiness, healing, and wholeness will be different.

While I believe this to be true, there is also a common thread among different faith practices that encourages us to find joy, meaning, and purpose in the service of others. Most major faith traditions—Christianity, Islam, and Judaism for example—emphasize that serving others is not only a moral duty but a sacred act that reflects the character of God or the higher self. Even in traditions like Buddhism and Hinduism, which focus more on enlightenment or unity with the divine, selfless service is seen as a path toward spiritual growth and liberation, helping one transcend ego and cultivate compassion. Many faiths teach that **when you give of yourself and your time, energy, and care, you not only uplift others, you also experience healing, perspective, and a sense of purpose.**

Think about it. It's difficult to be consumed with your own ruminations if you are earnestly and sincerely listening to someone answer how they're doing or volunteering with others to serve food at a soup kitchen.

Helping someone else puts your own struggles in a broader context. You begin to see that suffering is a shared human experience. You're not alone in your suffering. This can reduce feelings of isolation and self-pity. Our faith, no matter what that faith might be, teaches us that we're all part of something larger than ourselves. When you serve others, you step into that larger story. You're reminded that your life has purpose beyond your pain, which can be deeply grounding and healing. In fact, Gretchen Rubin also says in her *Secrets of Adulthood* book that "When in doubt about how to spend our time, energy or money, spend it on relationships." At its greatest, being of service is not just about meeting the needs of others—it's about embodying divine love and acknowledging the sacred worth of every person. It shifts the focus from the self to the community and transforms both the giver and the recipient.

Acts of kindness and service release positive chemicals in the brain, such as dopamine and oxytocin. These positive chemicals can ease anxiety, depression, and stress and essentially lift the emotional fog we sometimes get lost in. When we serve others, we are practicing trust in divine wisdom. Instead of being paralyzed by our own problems, we take a step in faith, believing that God or the Universe is still at work, even if our own circumstances aren't yet resolved.

Sometimes the Healing Action Is No Action at All

We will continue to experience the rainbow of emotions throughout our lifespan because that is the human experience. But here's the thing—it can be beautiful even when it's painful. My rabbi friend says the following:

> Embedded into the DNA of my faith is to lament, and the stories of our faith are about people crying out to God in pain. Sometimes that's the beginning seeds of our liberation and being able to live more fully. The seeds of awareness and wisdom that we are not alone and that we're not here forever and how we're going to make the most of this, to make the most of this time on Earth. My faith keeps me in a place to live more fully and connect more deeply.

The truth is, friends, that sometimes you just need to sit in your feelings. Ugh, I know. That sounds awful, doesn't it? Why do we need to sit in our feelings? Well, for one, we aren't robots. Crying out in pain is part of the human experience. Allowing ourselves to experience those feelings, both painful and pleasureful, is the beginning of our liberation. And for another, as my pastor brilliantly put it, "Jesus became human to feel all the things."

This is a good time to remember that this journey we've embarked on will not be perfect. You can be doing this work for decades and be an intuitive eating expert and still find yourself having an emotional eating experience. Perhaps it was using food as a reward for a bad day. Perhaps you were bored. Or perhaps you were trying to use food to numb out for a bit. Guess what? It's okay. You have done nothing wrong, and this says zero about who you are and your worth.

So what does sitting in your feelings even look like? It could look like a number of things, but the key is to work toward accepting the emotions versus trying to change or distract from them. That might be sitting and doing some breathing exercises or meditating. It could be journaling and writing out your thoughts and feelings on paper or in a digital diary. It could even be going outside and staring up at the sky, whether it's filled with stars or with clouds, and allowing yourself to be.

It may also be prayer. Prayer can look very different from person to person, but at its core, prayer is an intentional communication stemming from a desire to connect to something bigger than ourselves, be that God, the Universe, your higher power, or any other name. We can talk out loud and speak in our minds, or we can just sit in quiet contemplation with our feelings. We can ask for support, love, guidance, or strength. For billions of people, prayer can be helpful and sometimes even a lifeline. Prayer certainly doesn't always have to be about asking for something. Some of my most heartfelt prayers have been about expressing gratitude. Even in times of turbulence, expressing gratitude with sincerity and devotion has provided me with a deep sense of peace.

In the Islamic faith, Muslims are required to pray five times a day. As my colleague shared with me, this is actually self-care oriented. Muslims believe prayer helps us remember why we're here. It provides perspective and allows them to stay connected to God, seek guidance, and express gratitude. In Chapter 95, verses 5 and 6 of the Quran, it is said that "with hardship comes ease." The phrase emphasizes the importance of patience and perseverance during times of struggle. It provides a hope that God will eventually bring relief and that the hardship may even be an opportunity for spiritual growth and development. If I may borrow a phrase from one of my favorite people and brilliant eating disorder specialist colleague, "It's a gift." It's amazing how often and in how many different instances I've heard her use this expression. At its core, it reminds us that everything has a lesson behind it and offers not only something to learn, but also an opportunity for self-exploration and self-development.

If you ever have an emotional eating experience again, (spoiler alert, you will), take some time to reflect on the behavior. It's critically important that this self-reflection occurs without any self-criticism or judgment. Because again, you've done nothing wrong. Instead, pause and think to yourself, "What was going on for me today? It's a bit out of my routine to eat mindlessly, and I wasn't physically hungry. How have I been feeling today? Are there any feelings I am trying to avoid?" This kind of pause and reflection is gold for self-development and growth. If you find yourself getting stuck or having frequent emotional eating behaviors, it may be very beneficial to reach out to a clinician for support.

This may not surprise you, but the most common mental health disorders in the world are anxiety disorders. According to the World Health Organization (WHO), there are an estimated 284 million people suffering from anxiety disorders globally. I see this in my own inner circle of loved ones, myself included. Fortunately, there are a number of effective ways to cope, which we've already discussed. However, because the prevalence of anxiety is so high, allow me to share some relevant Bible verses I've come across that may be helpful as well.

- *Do not be anxious about anything, but in every situation, by prayer and petition, with thanksgiving, present your requests to God. And the peace of God, which transcends all understanding, will guard your hearts and your minds in Christ Jesus.* (Philippians 4:6-7)
- *Peace I leave with you; my peace I give you. I do not give it to you as the world gives. Do not let your hearts be troubled and do not be afraid.* (John 14:27)
- *So do not fear, for I am with you; do not be dismayed, for I am your God. I will strengthen you, I will help you; I will uphold you with my righteous hand.* (Isaiah 41:10)
- *The Lord is close to the brokenhearted and saves those who are crushed in spirit.* (Psalm 34:18)

And my personal favorite:

- *Be still and know that I am God.* (Psalm 46:10)

I am not a theologian or an expert on the Bible in any way, but something about this verse clicks for me. When the s**t hits the fan, and life is chaotic, and everything feels overwhelming and intolerable, reminding myself that the Universe has a plan is wildly comforting. There is a power higher than myself who loves me as a sacred part of the Universe.

Practice Coping with Your Emotions

How are you currently coping with all of life's stressors? What grounds you and brings you back into connection when you feel overwhelmed and distressed? Consider the moments when you have felt at peace. What was happening in those moments? You might also gently explore what emotions you hope food will soothe. Perhaps you long for comfort, steadiness, relief, distraction, or a sense of being cared for. When you reflect honestly on what food soothes for you and what it does not, you begin to see emotional eating with more compassion and less judgment. You start to recognize the deeper needs beneath the craving, especially the ones that are asking to be paid attention to and addressed with kindness.

Next, begin gathering a set of supportive coping tools that honor both your emotional life and your spirituality. Write out five to ten options that help you feel grounded and connected. Allow food to be one valid choice. Alongside it, include other options such as prayer, journaling, meditation, calling a friend, spending time in nature, listening to music, creating something with your hands, moving your body gently, or allowing yourself to rest. Some of the most useful skills to learn are breathing exercises. No matter where you are or what stressor you are facing, you always have your breath. Learning a skill such as box breathing can be extremely useful in times of high stress. (*Box breathing* is when you breathe in for four counts, hold your breath for four counts, exhale for four counts, and then hold your breath again for four counts before your next inhalation. You repeat this four times.) You can also add the 5-4-3-2-1 grounding skill to your list: Find five things you can see, four things you can touch, three things you can hear, two things you can smell, and one thing you can taste. This exercise is widely used in therapy and spiritual grounding practices because it reorients you to your body and to the present moment where you can respond rather than react. Overall, this technique becomes a map back to yourself, a reminder that comfort is available in many forms.

Finally, consider committing to one simple act of service this week. Send a kind message to someone on your mind. Check on a friend. Share a meal. Donate a small amount of your time to an organization whose values you support. Service reconnects you to compassion, purpose, and the understanding that we are all held to a greater connected purpose. In this way, tending to others becomes another way of tending to yourself and another way of remembering that love surrounds you and moves through you, even in difficult moments.

Chapter Nine

Respect Your Body and Have Reverence for Your Sacred Vessel

We have a live oak tree in our backyard. The tree is about twenty feet tall, and the base of it is maybe four feet in diameter. It's a big tree that's home to many different birds and squirrels and provides much-needed relief by shading our patio from the hot Texas summers with its canopy of evergreen leaves. Live oaks are the most common trees in Texas because of their hardiness and longevity. Despite being commonplace as part of the landscape of Texas, any time we have new guests over and they walk out into our backyard, they always say the same thing: "What a cool tree!" They say this because our tree is unique in that *it grows horizontally.*

When we first moved into the house, I was able to stand on my tiptoes and reach the largest branch with the ends of my fingers. Now I have to watch my head when I mow the lawn. The tree may eventually succumb to the weight of the branches seemingly growing in the wrong direction, but we are doing all we can each year to save it, including hiring an arborist who agrees that it is worth saving. It is simply too cool not to do so.

For many people, communing with nature is how they connect to spirituality. It may be hard to articulate how, but they can feel it, and nature is the vessel to get them there. Have you ever strolled the beach looking for shells? Sometimes the most amazing ones you find are ones that have unique colors and textures because they've been weathered by the salt and sand. Similarly, the lack of uniformity with wildflowers only serves to enhance their beauty. They are uneven, they don't match, they have no pattern or symmetry, and yet, we love to see this display of nature's design. None of these examples are perfect, and that's the point.

The variety of landscapes across the globe is spectacular. We can each find such beauty, inspiration, and awe in nature *even though it's far from perfect.* In fact, **nature is filled with examples of imperfection, which often makes it even more spectacular.** As I write this section of the book, it's autumn. The leaves are just beginning to change. Those leaves are actually dying, but their transformation is so beautiful that people wait all year for the colors of fall to adorn their communities. We seek out the imperfect beauty of nature.

We also feel spiritually connected to nature because it makes us feel closer to something bigger than ourselves. After all, in many spiritual traditions, the God who created the world also made us, and some of those traditions also say He literally made us from the same stuff. Even if you don't believe in an almighty creator, science confirms that we're made of the same material as the stars. However, we don't usually take that connection far enough. We don't take that final step of allowing ourselves to contain the same imperfections as nature, the same lack of symmetry, the same lack of an ideal. You see where I'm going. We expect just the opposite of ourselves. We do everything we can to fit into a normative standard of an ideal appearance.

What if we didn't?

What if we saw ourselves as we do leaves and trees and seashells? I very much like thinking of myself as a wildflower. I certainly know many women who are deserving of such a comparison. What if we allowed ourselves the same grace to be imperfect? What if we admired and celebrated that imperfect beauty instead of lamenting it? Instead of seeing it as a failure of our character? How much better would, well, everything be?

We now come to the principle of respecting your body. This can be one of the more challenging principles on this journey. Our end goal is a complete transformation in the perception of our bodies, a transformation that will return us to the idea that our bodies are sacred vessels that carry our souls. Yes, this means our bodies are essentially meat sacs. (And yes, I use this term in my professional practice.) And no, this doesn't mean you will suddenly have zero body image issues and instantly love the way your body looks. What it will mean, hopefully, is that you'll realize the way your body (or meat sac) looks just doesn't really matter. We're not meant to be perfect; we're meant to live wild, full, and loving journeys for as long as we're here.

When No Opinion Can Be a Good Feeling

The term "body positivity" has been part of the mainstream discourse about body image for a long time, but you may be less familiar with the terminology of "body neutrality." Eating disorder therapist Anne Poirier coined the phrase in 2015 to convey the idea of "prioritizing the body's function and what it can do rather than its appearance" to her clients. She wanted to move away from the idea of loving or hating your body and instead targeting a neutral stance. Many clinicians have since adopted the term "body neutrality" or "body acceptance" over the use of "body positivity" as it seems to resonate more with patients. For many people, loving your body just doesn't feel attainable. Whether for clinical reasons (such as people with eating disorders and body dysmorphia), trauma, medical issues, physical disabilities, or cultural reasons, having a neutral stance about your body often seems to be easier and more relatable for many individuals.

I recently attended an incredible workshop centered around the Asian American experience as it relates to eating disorders and body image. The presenter shared that there is tremendous pressure on Asian Americans to maintain an idealized thinness. In fact, in some Asian countries, the ideal is closer to what we might consider underweight in the United States. Comments about body changes and weight gain are common due to collectivist values around group belonging, making it socially acceptable for Aunt Susan to comment about the food you're eating and your waistline. Because of this, body positivity becomes even more difficult as it's not just society at large but your inner circles who impose these expectations.

In speaking with my colleague of the Islamic faith, she shared with me that even women who are covered from public view struggle with body image. She said that women are considered sacred and wear headscarves to help them focus on the beauty within and not on external beauty. However, the dissipation of Western diet culture over social media has negatively affected body image for women in societies even where they are completely covered and wearing garments designed to hide shape. As my colleague said, "Women who are covered head to toe are actually thought of as better and more God-like because they are being stricter about concealing their beauty. But yes, we absolutely still struggle with body image. We struggle with our egos like anyone else." Diet culture knows no bounds in the age of the Internet.

If it's bad for those of us who often fit societal norms, what about people in marginalized populations? One staggering statistic from the Trevor Project 2022 National Survey on LGBTQ Youth Mental Health found that 87 percent of LGBTQ youth reported being dissatisfied with their body, and 90 percent of transgender and nonbinary youth reported body dissatisfaction, with their primary reason being the difference between their biological sex and their gender identity. For this group especially, body positivity is an impossible goal. Even body neutrality or acceptance may seem difficult if the term is limited only to the feeling of neutrality. But if it's expanded into a broader sense, it can be therapeutic for many individuals across many groups and cultures.

One of my favorite ways to expand upon this is using language from PhD siblings Lindsay and Lexie Kite, authors of *More Than a Body: Your Body Is an Instrument, Not an Ornament*. This incredible book has a ton of great insight and research. My favorite quote comes from the book title: "Your body is an instrument, not an ornament." Another favorite comes from dietitian Kirsten Ackerman, who posted, "Body acceptance IS NOT about trying to like the rolls on your belly or the cellulite on your thighs. Body acceptance is about LIBERATING yourself from the idea that what your body looks like says a damn thing about your worth as a human being." Such brilliant gems.

These types of philosophies are the North Star of approaching a different way of looking at your body. They point a path toward respect and appreciation for what your body can do versus only how it looks. **When you think about it, our bodies can do some super cool stuff.** The human heart beats more than three billion times in an average lifespan. The human eye can distinguish thousands of different colors, and your nose can recognize thousands of different scents. Your skin is the body's largest organ and can be grafted from one part of your body to grow on another part. Human teeth are just as strong as shark teeth. And guess what? Being thin has nothing to do with any of these amazing functions. But sadly, instead of marveling at what our bodies can do, we get lost in pursuing diet culture ideals and standards of aesthetic beauty, no matter how unattainable.

And keep in mind that whatever society's standards for the ideal body type are today, they will be changing again soon anyway. And then again. And then again. In just the last hundred years, we've seen the body ideal go from an ultra-thin boyish figure to full curves but only in the "right" places to strong and fit and beyond.

This is not to say that men aren't also subject to body image issues and the pressures of an ideal body type. In fact, it is heartening to see more men speak about their body image issues and the struggles of feeling pressured to be as lean and muscular as possible. During a press conference, an actor who had undergone a superhero body transformation for a particular role spoke about his experiences with emotional eating, guilt and shame, and the difficulties of being caught in that cycle. His vulnerability in that moment illuminated the struggle that men also feel. This was all the more noteworthy because while he's not the only man to feel this way, he's certainly one of the few in Hollywood speaking out about it. In one of my favorite podcasts, *Ten Percent Happier,* American journalist Dan Harris had an incredible episode with intuitive eating co-founder Evelyn Tribole. In the episode, he was vulnerable and shared his own struggles with body image and his relationship to food. He described learning the principles of intuitive eating as "life changing." While these are only two public examples, there are certainly many more. And so I hope my male readers will not feel as if I have discounted their feelings or their experience. It is real.

Additionally, I'm also very aware that there are individuals who may possess society's version of the ideal body type yet feel they have been "skinny shamed" at times. This is also real. So let me be very clear: It is never okay to shame anyone about their body. Hard stop.

This is why the concept of body neutrality is so powerful. It interrupts the belief that your body must be evaluated in order for you to live your life. **Instead of asking you to love your body or hate it, body neutrality invites you to stop judging your body and to step out of the courtroom entirely.** It doesn't matter your gender, age, race, or any other aspect of your identity. Everyone is vulnerable to body image issues. Each of us can probably name at least one aspect of our bodies we wish looked differently. However, when that aesthetic desire is released and when we can remember that we're all sacred vessels (or meat sacs), our mental brain space clears out the shame and pressure and makes room for living your life.

Happiness Fits Like a Glove Every Time

When the coronavirus pandemic hit, I was already going through the totally stress-free experience of planning a wedding. Insert heart palpitation. I had to reschedule and cancel and reschedule and cancel and reschedule and cancel our wedding three times. On top of the fear and anxiety we were all feeling during this time, I also experienced added stress and repeated heartbreaking disappointment from navigating all of the vendors and guest travel. And then, of course, there was the situation with my dress.

There are only a handful of people who know what I'm about to share here. The truth is that the dress I wore on my wedding day was not the original dress I bought. When I bought my first wedding dress, I went with my mom to a modern boutique in downtown Dallas. We found THE dress, and I took the obligatory picture with my mom holding a sign that said, "She said Yes to the Dress." It was gorgeous. I felt beautiful. I could picture myself walking down the aisle to my fiancé in this one-of-a-kind designer, not inexpensive bridal gown. Except, as you already know, my wedding celebration was pushed back. And then pushed back again. And then again after that.

My now husband and I decided that despite the pandemic, he and I would still keep our original date. Because of the pandemic, it was only us and our pastors by the creek behind our church. We recorded the brief ceremony on our cell phone. Now let me say, that was still one of the single best days of my life. Marrying my husband was the smartest decision I have ever made, and when I think of that day, all I think about is how grateful and euphoric I felt. When I look at the photograph of us from that day, I look so in love. And I do think I look beautiful … in my jeans and white blouse. Because that is what I decided to wear that day. Because only three people would see me and the world was falling apart, the designer bridal gown did not feel appropriate. I also still believed someday I would get the chance to wear it in front of all of our friends and family when we could reschedule.

Although the day finally came when we rescheduled with our friends and family and repeated our vows with our pastors, I was not wearing the original gown, nor was I wearing the jeans and white blouse. Instead, I was wearing a new dress. I'd had to because the original dress no longer fit me.

I had gained some weight during the pandemic, and I was not alone. The National Institute of Health reported that 42 percent of Americans gained weight during the pandemic. While the majority of my mind and spirit wanted to (and did) rage against the weight-loss companies that took advantage of this and made people feel unfairly ashamed, there was a small but real part of me that struggled when I went back to the seamstress for my final fitting and my dress no longer looked the same on me.

I had brought my sister with me. I watched her watching me, waiting for me to be the smiling blushing bride in the three-way mirror. But I couldn't do it. I felt unattractive. I felt disappointed. And then more than anything else, I felt like an absolute hypocrite.

How could I spend my life's work telling people that your weight does not define your worth and then feel terrible about my reflection as it looked back at me that day? I had spent years overcoming body image dissatisfaction and had completely embraced a body neutral stance. And boom. In one day, it's gone?

I felt like such a fraud.

I tumbled down a shame spiral that resulted in tears as soon as I left the fitting and got into my car. I told my sister some of the truth that day, and she listened and was supportive. I couldn't even articulate at that moment how I felt. But as awful as I felt that afternoon, my pride in myself for what happened next outshines that uncomfortable memory.

I let myself be sad for the rest of the day. Then I made two decisions. One, I would recognize the truth that no one is perfect, and that despite my extensive work in this space, I still lived in a diet-culture, thin-idealist society that believed brides should look a certain way. I could have a brief setback and then get back on track and stick to my values and forgive myself for the normal period of doubts. It didn't make me a fraud. It made me human. Two, I would not try and lose weight to get back into the dress. Instead, I would buy a new dress. And I did.

I went to a bridal dress chain store and bought a very inexpensive dress off the rack that required almost no alterations. I doubled down on my now curvier body and chose a dress that hugged me head to toe. And you know what? When I finally had my wedding day, I looked and felt like a total bombshell. I had not given into diet culture. I had not tried to do some crazy crash diet. I had returned to what I know to be true: my weight does not define me. My inner circle loves me, and my appearance doesn't matter. My family loves me no matter what. My husband loves me no matter what. God loves me no matter what. *And I have sacred worth no matter what.* We *all* do.

What is sacred worth? The Bible says that all people are created in God's image: "So God created man in his own image." (Genesis 1:27) Therefore, **our sacred worth means that we all have intrinsic and inherent value.** So when I look at the pictures of that day, all I feel is gratitude.

I share this story because coming to a place of body neutrality is not a perfect path. You can be ten years in and still have a day where you get sucked back into the lies of diet culture. It's okay. It's not your fault. But also, there is so much power and strength when you can say "eff diet culture" and refuse to give in, when you not only embrace who you are but celebrate the heck out of it. As Rumi said, "Know then that the body is merely a garment, go seek the wearer, not the cloak."

Some Thoughts on Medication, Surgically-Induced Weight Loss, and the Body

We've seen slightly more diversity in the body types of celebrities over the past decade, largely due to the body positivity and inclusivity trends that many of these celebrities have championed on social media. Although, at the time of this writing, that is changing as well. Some of the most vocal body-positive celebrities have made the choice—and it is their choice—to take weight-loss drugs to alter their body types. A quick search on the Internet will give you dozens of well-known names that have jumped on the GLP-1 bandwagon. The truth is, because the prevalence of those drugs is so dramatically high, there is a strong likelihood that this book makes it into the hands of someone on those medications. Currently, an estimated 15 million Americans are taking a GLP-1 drug, and 30 million people have reported trying them. That's a lot of people.

I have two thoughts on this subject. Okay, that's not true; I have several. But for the purposes of this book, I will share two of them. First, and most importantly, your body is none of my business. Your body is not the business of Congress. Your body is not the business of your Aunt Susan. Your body is no one's business but your own. Take a weight-loss drug, pierce your eyebrow, tattoo your whole back, get calf implants, have a face lift. It is no one's business. It is your body and your choice, and I will champion your right to body autonomy until my dying day.

Second, as a clinician, I have been trained and believe deeply in the concept of providing informed consent. What does that mean? For most people, it's one of those pesky papers in a stack of admissions forms you have to fill out when you see a new healthcare provider. For myself and my colleagues, it is a way to ensure that we have provided a patient with sufficient information so they are completely aware of both the potential benefits and potential risks of a proposed treatment.

I have low confidence that there is sufficient informed consent for patients seeking GLP-1s for the purpose of weight loss. The Medical Students for Size Inclusivity created a brilliant GLP-1 Agonist Informed Consent Project that I highly recommend reviewing because most people are not provided a thorough overview regarding the risks of these medications. As not everyone is aware of how much misinformation there is within diet culture, many people are still under the mistaken belief that being thinner equals being healthier, including much of the medical community. As such, patients can justify wanting these medications without any medical conditions, and doctors may gladly prescribe them because they will be "for the patient's health." To be clear, I place zero shame or blame on individuals in this situation. We all coexist in this fat-phobic diet culture together. But again, there is a lack of honest and transparent informed consent.

Take, for example, how the marketing around these drugs addresses "food noise." In general, this marketing claims that the mental chatter in our minds about food and cravings is a symptom these drugs can cure. However, myself and the clinicians in this field know that 99 percent of the time, "food noise" is a direct result of restriction. If you are hungry, you will think of food. If you are depriving yourself of a specific type of food, you will crave it. It really is that simple. And we *want* our body sending us these signals. We *need* our brains to send us the cues that we *need* to eat. Marketing food noise as a problem is just more of diet culture and smart pharmaceutical advertising. The deeper question is not that we think about food, but why those thoughts feel so charged or uncomfortable. See Chapters 4 through 7 if you want to read about it again.

There's no question that these drugs can be incredibly helpful for diabetes, which is what they were originally designed for. In fact, "helpful" may be underselling it. GLP-1 can be life saving for people with *critically high A1C levels*. The research is clear on this. The research is less clear on the non-diabetic population. They're just still too new.

We do not yet have any good long-term data on the potential risks of these drugs.

For the severely diabetic population, the benefits outweigh the physical and mental health risks of GLP-1 drugs. But for those who are seeking smaller body types for purely aesthetic reasons, we can't possibly provide sufficient informed consent without long-term research. So far, short-term research has shown a host of digestive issues including nausea, vomiting, and diarrhea. Serious risks include pancreatitis, gastroparesis, bowel obstruction, gallbladder problems, and kidney problems. From a mental health perspective, risks include increased anxiety, depression, and even suicidality. As clinicians, we have an ethical responsibility to share our concerns and potential risks when someone wants to take a weight-loss drug that essentially creates what some providers consider medically-induced starvation.

We also know that some medical providers have prescribed the medication to patients who are already restricting. Atypical anorexia, which is an anorexic diagnosis for a body type that is not considered underweight, is severely underdiagnosed. Providers have an ethical responsibility to complete appropriate screenings for these medications; however, if the patient sitting in their exam room doesn't appear to have the stereotypical underweight body type, the likelihood is that an eating disorder may be overlooked, especially because less than six percent of individuals with an eating disorder actually have an underweight body type, despite the stereotype.

I also have low confidence that there is adequately communicated informed consent on what happens when a non-diabetic patient goes off of these drugs. Many people are unable to tolerate the side effects or they reach their desired weight and don't like the idea of being on medication for the rest of their lives. For many others, it becomes cost-prohibitive. So patients stop taking them, with or without the knowledge of their healthcare providers, with varied results. Yet, like with any weight-loss venture, we're finding that much, if not all, of the weight lost returns. At this point, people become understandably discouraged and may go back on the medication with some choosing to commit for the long haul. Moreover, many people start exhibiting eating disorder behaviors after discontinuing the medications in an effort to maintain the weight loss, even if they never had eating disorder behaviors in the past.

(Can you see where this is going? We have the potential again for weight cycling. As discussed in Chapter 2, there are significant physical and mental health risks associated with weight cycling.)

Combine the lack of long-term research, the bias of many medical professionals against people in larger bodies, and the misinformation about obesity as a disease, and you have a recipe for overprescription and overuse of these drugs well beyond their initial intention and design.

Although weight loss surgery has declined, notably as weight loss drugs have increased, it's still worth addressing. Bariatric surgery historically dominated the weight loss treatment plans for people in larger bodies, and as more long term research is coming out, we see more risks associated with it, including complications from the surgery, gastrointestinal (GI) issues, alcohol disorders, and increased anxiety, depression, and suicidality.

In my conversations with others, people seem to expect GI issues with weight-loss drugs, treatments, and surgeries, but they are often surprised by the mental health side effects. Those of us in the behavioral healthcare landscape, particularly those with eating disorder expertise, have zero surprise. For people who hate their bodies, no amount of manipulation to their bodies will suddenly uncover the secret to everlasting happiness. Why? Because life is hard! The human experience includes pain, loss, stress, grief, and trauma. **It is a heart-crushing reality for people who des-**

perately believed that if only they were thin, then everything would be okay only to find out everything just isn't.

Those of us who work in the eating disorder and therapy spaces, know it's never really about your body. Body image struggles are the symptom, not the cause. Lasting happiness comes with living your values and finding and intentionally investing in connection. The alternative is constantly manipulating a body that will change, decline, and age no matter how much we fight against it. When you're eighty years old, you will not look like you did when you were twenty, no matter how many products you use or how much surgery you get. And you shouldn't be made to feel that you must.

In the Emmy award-winning show *Fleabag,* there is a memorable scene in the first episode featuring the title character, Fleabag, and her sister Claire. The two women are attending a feminist lecture together, and the speaker begins by saying, "Please raise your hands if you would give up five years of your life for the so-called 'perfect body.'" While the rest of the audience remains still, both Fleabag's and Claire's hands shoot up in the air. After looking around and realizing they were the only ones to do so and that it was likely not the answer the speaker was attempting to solicit, Claire leans over and whispers, "We are bad feminists."

In reality, Fleabag and Claire are far from alone in this sentiment. A UK study found that 30 percent of women would trade at least one year of their life to achieve their ideal body weight and shape. The sample was taken from women at multiple universities in the UK. These young, ambitious, bright women who have their whole lives before them would shave off a year to achieve this. Some participants said they would trade as much as ten years. Let that sink in. I think there is a clear argument that the impact of poor body image is not just a cosmetic concern. It's a serious public health and mental health issue that affects how people view themselves, value their lives, and make life choices.

Everyone of every gender deserves to feel and believe that they are worthy of love, dignity, and respect regardless of their size, shape, and looks. **We need to view how our bodies change as we age as a privilege, not a consequence. Our wrinkles and stretch marks are earned through our lived experiences.** Our beautiful sacred vessels that carry us and evolve with us from birth are worth celebrating. Aging is a gift for each of us. After all, consider the alternative.

The Gift of Self-Acceptance

In Buddhist philosophy, one of the three universal truths is Impermanence or *Anicca*. In its simplest explanation, it means that nothing lasts forever. The concept is that everything is constantly changing and in constant motion—the weather, our relationships, our emotions, the seasons, and yes, the aging of our bodies. When we fight against these changes and cling to what we have no control over, this leads to suffering or the second universal truth known as *Dukkha*. The third universal truth, non-self or *Anatta,* is a bit more complex. At its heart, Anatta aims to release us from this suffering by transitioning from clinging to a sense of self or identity to recognizing that we are constantly in flow and not a fixed object. We shift from "Who am I?" to "How am I connected?"

The late Elisabeth Kubler-Ross, one of the world's most renowned experts on grief and loss, stated, "It is not the end of the physical body that should worry us. Rather, our concern must be to live while we're alive—to release our inner selves from the spiritual death that comes with living behind a facade designed to conform to external definitions of who and what we are." Kubler-Ross is reminding us that spiritual life is not defined by how long our physical bodies last and that we lose the authenticity of our lives when we hide behind masks or live only to meet others' expectations. In intuitive eating, **respecting your body means honoring it as it is right now and valuing dignity, self-compassion, and authenticity over unrealistic expectations.**

This perspective aligns closely within Buddhism. The body is not judged as good or bad but observed with kindness and curiosity. Suffering is understood to arise from craving, aversion, and comparison, which includes striving for a "better" body. Buddhist teaching encourages practices that emphasize acceptance of what is rather than trying to control it and radical self-compassion without attachment. The body is seen as impermanent. It changes moment by moment, and therefore is not a reliable container for identity or worth. In Buddhism, when we stop demanding that the body be different in order for us to be at peace, we create space for dignity and freedom right now.

When I was going through my yoga teacher certification, we learned a great deal about the Yoga Sutras. *Sutra* comes from the Sanskrit word for "thread," and each sutra offers a thread of insight through study, reflection, and lived practice. In Hindu philosophy, *ahimsa,* or non-harm in the Yoga Sutras, is named first among the *yamas,* the ethical foundations of yoga. Ahimsa emphasizes a profound spiritual framework for understanding what it means to respect the body. While ahimsa is often associated with nonviolence toward others, animals, and the Earth, its most intimate application is nonviolence toward oneself. When the body is treated as an enemy to be conquered rather than a sacred expression of life, ahimsa is broken not through malice but through conditioning. Seen through ahimsa, respecting the body is not about achieving a certain appearance or health status. It is about reducing harm and increasing care and reverence for the body that is a sacred vehicle for the soul.

In all my years of clinical practice, research, and in my personal life, I have never met anyone who had a positive outcome from hating their body. Most people seem to hate or feel disgust toward their bodies or parts of their bodies. And yet, if you logically tell someone in this frame of mind that this is a losing battle, they won't agree. In fact, they may believe that if only they could be even less tolerant of their imperfect bodies, they could find the willpower and motivation to work harder. Not only will this not work, but it's certainly not what God wants for us.

The movement of the weight-loss industry toward weight-loss medications, specifically GLP-1 drugs, is still evolving. This drug has already dramatically changed the industry landscape in just the last year, and I think it's reasonable to assume that it will look different next year and five years from now as we learn more. One final note on these medications: At the time of this writing, they are a hot topic. Moreover, the National Alliance of Eating Disorders reported that its helpline had its busiest day ever after an ad for GLP-1 was marketed during the third quarter of the 2024 Super Bowl.

I respect (as should we all) anyone's right to make individual health choices for their body. Whether you're diabetic or not, if you've made the choice to take a GLP-1, no one has any right to shame you for your choices. I also respect (as should we all) that there are still millions of people living in larger bodies who are under tremendous pressure from society's anti-fat bias to take these drugs even when they have no underlying medical conditions. They deserve our compassion and support, not our judgment.

In 2015, the Association for Size Diversity and Health (ASDAH) created an incredible animated video called "The Problem with Poodle Science." It's available online and is a must-watch. The video positions the poodle as the ideal dog standard in terms of size and shape. It then asks the viewer to imagine comparing all dogs to poodles. By doing this, it cleverly posits the question, "How could a mastiff or a chihuahua ever have the same size and shape as a poodle?" The analogy is clear—when the same logic is applied to humans, we can see the inherent weight stigma and flawed research.

It is almost impossible not to compare ourselves when we are constantly surrounded by curated images, filters, and loud cultural messages about how bodies are "supposed" to look (remember

Chapter 2?). But **comparison steals joy every single time,** and it harms bodies of all sizes. One of the best tips I can provide is to stop comparing by noticing when you're doing it and actively reminding yourself to *let that sh*t go.* Comparing bodies is like comparing poodles to mastiffs, as the ASDAH argues. Diversity is not a flaw—it is the design! Just like our height or shoe size, bodies are meant to come in a wide range of shapes, structures, and expressions. There is no single "right" way to look. Remembering that truth can be deeply freeing.

If you worry that people may see changes in your body shape and size as "letting yourself go," take a page out of Registered Dietician Alissa Rumsey's book, *Unapologetic Eating: Make Peace with Food and Transform Your Life,* and tell yourself , "Yes, you have let yourself go. You've let yourself go do other things rather than worrying about your body or food all of the time. You've let yourself go do more creative, meaningful, joyful things. You've let yourself go be powerful, content and unapologetic."

God doesn't want us to waste our time on feeling shame, guilt, and self-disparagement related to our bodies. I promise you He does not care about our jeans size, and He doesn't want you to either. He has bigger things to worry about, and so do we. **Our bodies are miraculous creations of the Universe.** They are the vessels of the divine.

If after all of this you're still struggling with body image, don't stress. You're not alone, especially if this is your first time reflecting on some of these points. I've worked with patients who have been doing this work for years and still struggle at times. I've already admitted I have, too. Even for people who have lived these principles for years, seeing photographs of themselves can cause struggles with body image, whether it's seeing old pictures and lamenting the body they once had or seeing a recent picture and struggling with the image portrayed. But you need to remember something. You know how you'll take a picture of a beautiful sunset or a gorgeous landscape but it never does it justice? The same is true for you, my friend. You are that beautiful sunset, and the best camera in the world can't capture what it's like to be in your presence.

Giving up on trying to obtain the "thin ideal" is a noble cause with innumerable benefits, but it also comes with a potential grieving process. There is the loss of the younger version of your body and the loss that what you've worked so hard to accomplish for years may never happen. That's a lot to process. But oh, the other side of that grief is so beautiful, and there is infinitely more to gain than what you perceive to have lost.

Practice Respecting Your Body

This is a particularly challenging chapter for many. When you've been focusing on trying to change your body for most of your life, pivoting towards acceptance and respect can feel like a really big leap. Nature can help. Pay attention to the breathtaking imperfections in nature, such as the beauty in a crooked tree or the shifting colors of a sunset. Then ask yourself why it feels so much harder to extend that same grace to your own body, which is also part of creation with all its perceived imperfections.

Consider journaling about what the phrase "sacred worth" means to you. Does your current self-worth reflect that truth, or has it become tied to your weight, shape, and appearance even in subtle ways? Your body was never meant to be a project or a proof of value. You were created with inherent dignity. When you imagine believing wholeheartedly that your worth is God-given and unchanging, consider how that belief might transform the way you speak to yourself, the way you choose clothing, the way you nourish and rest, and the way you move through the world.

Here's the thing—**honoring the sacredness of your body is not one single moment but a lifelong practice.** You can begin gently. Take one piece of clothing that no longer feels good on your body and start a donation pile. When you have a few items, take it to your local donation center and let it go. Next, find something that fits your here-and-now body and reflects who you are today. This is not a failure. Choosing peace of mind is a success. Let it be an act of reverence rather than resignation.

You might also create a simple affirmation that roots you in spiritual truth. You may say something like, "My body is a sacred vessel of the divine. Its worth is inherent and cannot be earned. I honor it with compassion, dignity, and truth." Or find another statement that resonates more deeply with you in your own words. Read it aloud each morning for a week and notice how your spirit responds.

Respecting your body is ultimately an invitation to return to the truth that you were made in love and for love. When you treat your body with tenderness and respect, you are aligning yourself with that truth.

Chapter Ten

Move with Harmony and Flow of Body, Mind, and Spirit

If you would've told me twenty years ago that running was my joyful movement, I would've laughed in your face. Up until my late twenties, I had never run more than a mile in my life. And by run a mile, I mean walk/run begrudgingly in gym class. Then one day, a close friend of mine at the time who was also a distance runner told me the secret: "Go slower." She said to go as slow as possible to just get used to not stopping to walk. So I tried it. Truthfully, any power walker worth their salt would be speeding by my turtle like slow runs. But eventually going super slow increased my distance. One mile, two miles, three miles and then a 5K race. And guess what? Like anything else in life, it just took practice.

I think what I loved about it so much, and still do, is that one, it's free, and my inherited frugal genes are a sucker for "free;" two, it got me outside; three, it helped to ground me, get me out in nature, give me a different perspective. It helped to clear my mind or work stuff out. But, four, it also gives me an opportunity to commune with God.

My run might not start out in reverent contemplation. It may start out with thinking about work or my to-do list. I might initially be focused on the podcast I'm listening to or the drumming groove of whatever song is playing. But at some point, every time, there will come a moment when I have this feeling. It's actually hard to even put this into words. But there is always a moment when I feel connected to something more, something bigger. Something endlessly more important than whatever was previously on my mind.

Sometimes it's triggered by a perfect breeze, or I notice how green the trees have become from the last rain, or I see a bright red cardinal that stands out against the haze. Oftentimes it's as simple as looking up. I notice the bright blue sky or the sun peeking out from behind the clouds. Sometimes it's not even external. It's a moment where my heart is pounding, and I take a deep breath and I just feel ALIVE. That moment is almost always instantly transitioned to a feeling of intense gratitude. I feel something more. I feel God.

I can tell you with sincerity, never did I ever have an experience even remotely like that when I was in my twenties and forcing myself to exercise in a way I hated but felt compelled to do in order to burn the most calories.

By the time I hit my mid-thirties, I ran my first half marathon—a seeming impossibility only a few years earlier. But there is something about pushing yourself past your own self-imposed limitations that is freeing. Fast forward to present day, and I have run twelve half marathons and a full marathon, which is 26.2 miles. That you run. With your body!

What does it mean to find your joyful movement? It means finding the way to move your body that (no surprise here) brings you joy! Have you even found it yet? I find when I ask most people this question, they are stumped at first. They can tell you how they get their "exercise," but what is their joyful movement?

Deer in headlights. Allow me to start you on the journey with the greatest gift I can give you: Is there a particular type of exercise that you just hate and dread doing? STOP DOING IT.

There! I release you from your self-imposed shackles. Hate the elliptical? Stop doing it. Hate burpees? Stop doing them. Hate Pilates? Stop going. You are FREE! And listen closely, friends, because this next part is important: **Moving in a way that brings you joy is beautiful and helps return you to feeling gratitude for what your body can do.** Gratitude for the moment you are in. Gratitude for the joy in life especially during hard times. And gratitude for your higher power, whatever that may be. Who knows where it will take you!

When We Forget How to Move With Joy

Back in Chapter 4, I talked about Joey, *Friends,* and making peace with food. Here, I'll tell you about the characters Phoebe and Rachel and joyful movement. In one memorable episode of *Friends,* Phoebe and Rachel decide to go for a run together. After they arrive in Central Park, Rachel becomes immediately horrified at the way Phoebe runs—with her arms and legs flailing chaotically as she sprints. Rachel describes the movement as "a cross between Kermit the Frog and the Six Million Dollar Man." Later, when Rachel later confronts Phoebe about her embarrassment, Phoebe isn't the slightest bit deterred or defensive. Instead Phoebe says she runs, "...like she's free because it's the only way it's fun." She then asks Rachel if she remembers being a kid and running so fast towards the swings that she felt her legs would fall off but Rachel is still skeptical. However, the next time Rachel goes out for a run, she decides to give it a try and realizes she feels "great" and "so free and so graceful." The smile on her face and carefree demeanor illustrate how running has shifted from her exercise to her joyful movement.

In all seriousness, though, Phoebe makes a great point. Can we remember what it was like to be a kid and the way we played, finding endless ways to move our bodies? As a Gen X kid, I grew up in the era of parents wanting kids out of the house until the streetlights came on at night. We stayed outside and played games and used our imaginations. We climbed trees and rode our bikes and played flashlight tag. It was the best. What a time to be a kid! We came home dirty and maybe a little smelly, but we were also exhausted from the hours and hours of joyful movement with our friends and siblings. At what point did our attitude toward movement shift from joy to obligation? At what point did movement for play and fun transition to exercise for calorie burning? We may have all been different ages when that transformation happened, but it was likely a result of the same cause. And, of course, that cause is diet culture.

On my personal timeline, even when movement started to slightly shift towards "exercise," it was still somewhat fun. While the era of aerobics in the 1980s and 1990s, Jane Fonda and Billy Blanks, was definitely about burning calories and changing the shape of the body, it was still fun at times. *Sweatin' to the Oldies with Richard Simmons* could also be enjoyable as you did simple aerobic choreography to songs like "Dancing in the Street" or "Great Balls of Fire." But then in 2004, a reality TV show called, *The Biggest Loser,* premiered, and captured our attention in the worst, diet culture voyeuristic ways: We now had a front row seat to a new definition of exercise and not a single moment of it was joyful.

If you've never had the misfortune of watching this show, it was essentially a weight loss competition. People in larger bodies would compete against each other to see who could lose the most weight. The episodes consisted of watching the contestants restrict their food and exercise to the point of exhaustion and vomiting, all while being bullied and verbally abused by their "coaches." The cruelty and mistreatment was appalling. And millions of us tuned in.

There are many reasons why this show was objectively harmful, not only for the contestants but also the viewers. And high on that list of reasons was that it sold a lie about weight loss. In fact, a 2016 article in *The New York Times* reported on a study that National Institute of Health (NIH) researchers had conducted on former contestants of the show. Of the fourteen participants studied, on average, thirteen of them had gained back two-thirds of the weight they'd lost on the show, and five of them had gained back more than they'd lost. Their rapid and extreme weight loss resulted in a resting metabolic rate that remained severely suppressed even years after the show, making weight maintenance extraordinarily difficult.

However, this show also cast exercise as a necessary painful, even tortuous, method to achieve desired outcomes. It framed exercise as punishment. It promoted dangerous and unrealistic goals and eroded any intrinsic motivation for movement. All of a sudden it was normal to be told, "Don't stop until you drop," which of course can have multiple physical consequences on the body. But it wasn't just physical safety at risk. When exercise is consistently associated with humiliation, public weigh-ins, and body shaming, it becomes emotionally unsafe. People will inevitably come to associate movement with anxiety, dread, or self-criticism.

Movement isn't supposed to be like this. Like feasting, movement is celebration for what the body can do. It's meditation. It's communing with the Universe. It's summer time freedom. It's running so fast that we feel like our legs will come off, and, wow, how fun is that?

So what if we could repair our relationship with movement? What if we got back to how we moved as kids?

That Time I Ran a Marathon

Sometime after running a half-marathon or two, I got the itch, like most runners do, to tackle *the full marathon.* And I'm sincerely glad I did. I learned many things about myself during that training process and the race itself, including what my body is capable of with training and commitment. I also learned what my body is not capable of and it is not capable of running a marathon on the same fuel that it ran on for a half marathon. Common sense you say? Well, it honestly hadn't occurred to me until one day I was doing an 18-mile training run.

I finished the run in tears because I was so discouraged. I was winded. I was in pain. I hit the proverbial wall as they say. I remember saying to my friends who met me at the end that for a million dollars I could not have run eight more miles if it was marathon race day. I questioned whether or not I should even run the race. But then I thought, I might not be motivated by a million dollars, but I would do it for a sandwich... and that's when I realized, I was hungry!

The meal I ate before the run and the snacks I ate during the run were completely insufficient for the amount of calories I was burning. I needed more fuel! On my next training run, I ate accordingly and packed the calories I needed to sustain me. It was a game changer.

Now I will share without any shame at all that I will never run a full marathon again. However, I'm so glad I did it. It still makes me feel like a badass. But I 100 percent lost some of the joy I feel running when I was training for that race. And guess what? I don't have to. It's my choice because it's my joyful movement. 26.2 miles ain't joyful to me, and so I still run two to three times a week. Why? Because I love it. Because it is the single best thing I have found that prevents my anxiety from escalating during the week. Because my only competition is myself. Because it keeps my good cholesterol high to combat the bad cholesterol that my genetics keep high. And most importantly, because it brings me joy and makes me feel connected to something more.

Moving for Life, With Life

I had a brilliant therapist when I was in my twenties who gave me some of the best advice I've ever received. A simple two words. I still use it today if I'm having a hard time. Her advice: "Get up."

Get up and do what? you may wonder. That part was up to me. But the point was that when we feel low and stuck, interestingly, we put our bodies into positions that are also low and stuck. We stay in bed or glued to the couch. The intention of "get up" was to get unstuck physically with the hope that it would lead toward feeling unstuck emotionally. This has worked for me countless times in a variety of ways.

Why does this work? Right off the bat, standing or walking increases circulation, which can make you feel more alert, energized, and mentally clear. Physical action helps redirect your focus, giving your mind something constructive with which to engage. **Getting up and moving improves mood and well-being through neurochemical boosts, physical stimulation, and psychological shifts.** It's one of the fastest and most accessible ways to support mental health and break low-energy or low-mood states. Even small tasks (like making the bed, walking outside, or organizing a drawer) can provide a quick dopamine reward from achieving something. And we want that dopamine boost.

Dopamine is a neurotransmitter, or a chemical messenger, in the brain that plays a vital role in motivation, reward, pleasure, and movement. It helps create feelings of enjoyment and satisfaction and is also involved in learning, attention, and regulating emotions. When dopamine levels are balanced, we feel motivated and focused. When you engage in physical activity, your brain increases the production and release of dopamine.

Physical activity also enhances the sensitivity of dopamine receptors, meaning your brain becomes more responsive to the dopamine it produces. Over time, regular movement can even increase the availability of dopamine by promoting the growth of new neurons and supporting healthy brain chemistry. In other words, movement acts like a natural dopamine booster. It helps you feel more motivated, focused, and emotionally balanced.

What's extra cool is that the impact is both immediate and continues long term.

The biggest shift I'd love to encourage you to make is to get away from the very limited thinking of movement that diet culture has sold you, which is that movement equals exercise for the purpose of weight loss or weight "management." In reality, **movement is essential for holistic mind, body, and spiritual well-being.**

Physical activity benefits nearly every major system in the body, making it one of the most powerful tools for overall health. It strengthens the heart muscle, lowering resting heart rate, lowering blood pressure, lowering cholesterol and increasing circulation. It increases muscle and bone density. It strengthens lung capacity. It regulates hormones. It enhances cognitive function, focus and learning. And yes, it may (or may not) impact your weight.

If it doesn't impact your weight, that's okay! It's so important not to give up. Stay active. Find your joyful movement. The benefits are too great to ignore. You are also demonstrating a commitment to your health and doing so much good for your body even if you can not see the proof on the outside.

In my experience as a person and a therapist, I find that when people begin incorporating more movement into their lives, they tend to do the thing we all do, and they search for information about the best exercise to do for health. They look outside of themselves for recommendations. I get it. There's always a new study circulating about a different way to lift weights or a new kind of aerobic exercise for longevity, but don't give in to this impulse. For five years, I worked for Fitbit and then Google as a Senior Clinical Specialist from 2018 to 2023, and during this time, everyone was becoming obsessed with counting their steps, specifically to 10,000. You've heard that we're all supposed to get 10,000 steps a day, right? Have you ever asked where this number comes from?

Leading up to the 1964 Tokyo Olympics (that's right, 1964),

a Japanese company called Yamasa launched one of the first pedometers. They named it *manpo-kei,* which translates to "10,000 steps meter." Interestingly, this number wasn't selected because of any scientific research, but it was catchy and memorable. All that to say, now there is research that supports the benefits of getting your steps in each day. But the truth is that it doesn't require 10,000 steps to obtain those benefits. A large meta analysis in 2023 reviewed seventeen studies that included 226,000 participants. The findings showed that even modest step counts (around 2,300–4,000 steps per day) were linked with reduced risk compared with very low activity, and each additional increment of steps was associated with incremental health benefits. In other words, although higher step counts are attributed to positive health outcomes, substantial benefits begin at levels far below the traditional 10,000-step goal. So, yes, get those steps in, but don't drive yourself bananas with hitting a specific number, and certainly do it however you want. Don't get caught up in the numbers game, especially in the beginning of starting something new—number of sets, number of reps, number of minutes, etc.

Those things are great if you're trying to hit specific athletic or performance goals. But if you're trying to learn to listen to how your body feels and learn how to enjoy movement, then those numbers will function as rules and not serve the purpose of joyful movement. For example, a goal may be that you will go for a walk with your friend or partner twice a week with no predetermined time or distance goal. Another goal may be that whenever you move this week, you will journal afterwards how it made you feel.

There is also no shortage of ways to combine movement with spiritual pursuits. In a good mood and feeling like dancing? Maybe dance to some high energy gospel music. Feeling tense and anxious and need to stretch and reset? Try some breath focused yoga where every inhale is letting in the light and every exhale is letting go of the dark. Don't have anyone to walk with? Listen to a podcast of a spiritual advisor you enjoy.

If podcasts aren't your thing you can try a walking meditation, which is a form of mindfulness practice found in many Buddhist traditions. Instead of sitting still as in traditional meditation, you bring the same focused attention to the act of walking in order to bring the body, breath, and mind into harmony. You begin by choosing a short path of about 10 to 30 steps either in or outdoors. Then take a moment to pause, breathe, and set an intention. Thich Nhat Hanh, a modern Buddhist teacher, often said, "Walk as if you are kissing the Earth with your feet." As you walk, move slowly and pay attention to the feeling of lifting your foot, moving it forward, and placing it down. You can also try to match your steps with your breath by lifting your foot as you inhale and placing it down as you exhale. When you come to the end, pause, turn softly, and continue with the same calm awareness in your steps. Some people also find it helpful to silently repeat gentle phrases, like "lifting… moving… placing," or as Thich Nhat Hanh taught, "I have arrived… I am home."

The research is clear. The single best form of exercise that you can do for your body is… Wait for it… Are you leaning in? Are you ready? Here we go…

The single best form of exercise that you can do for your body is the one that you will do consistently.

Boom. There it is. A truth bomb laid at your feet. Despite the endless products out there that tell you their way and their product is the best, it's simply not true. If it feels like a burden, and you don't enjoy it, you will quit doing it. Everyone does.

The solution is to find your joyful movement that you will do consistently and regularly and never feels like a burden or an obligation, and on the contrary, is something you look forward to and that brings you joy and happiness. It's something you will never give up on. Instead you will have a regular schedule of movement that organically fits into your routine, getting you the movement that your physical, mental, and spiritual health craves.

It can be simple. Maybe every morning before work, you take

your dog on a walk or play fetch or keep away with them in your yard. You'll get your heart rate up, and there aren't many things more joyful than watching your pup's ears flop up and down while they walk on a leash or run back to you with their favorite ball. Perhaps you turn on your favorite music while you are preparing dinner each night and dance around your kitchen. I feel like God and the Universe would look down and smile at that image. As Kevin Bacon's character Ren McCormick in *Footloose* reminded us, it says in Psalms 149:3, "Let them praise His name with dancing."

So what is it for you? Friends, there are so many options! Perhaps you need to test out a few. Here are some examples for you to try:

- Walking
- Gardening
- Yoga
- Hiking
- Taking a beginner dance class
- Weight lifting
- Crossfit
- Tai Chi
- Rock climbing
- Swimming
- Martial arts
- And more!

You also don't have to stick to just one activity. Winston Churchill said, "To be really happy and really safe, one ought to have at least two or three hobbies, and they must all be real." I think the same rules apply here. I switch up my running with weight lifting and yoga. Both of those activities help my running, and most importantly, I enjoy them. For me they are real in that they authentically bring joy and positive energy into my life.

I received my yoga certification in the Sivananda discipline, which is a classic yoga based on the teachings of Swami Sivananda, a renowned Indian spiritual teacher and physician. In my classes, we learned that the *asanas,* or yoga poses, were part of an otherwise very spiritual practice to build muscle, flexibility, and endurance so that a practitioner could tolerate spending long hours sitting in meditation. We learned how to do the poses, of course. But a lot of our training was dedicated to the spiritual teachings of traditional yoga philosophy, much of which comes from a Hindu faith and cultural background. In fact, the last moment of most yoga classes ends with hands in a prayer position, a bowed head, and stating the word *namaste,* meaning, "The light (or the divine) within me sees and honors the light (or the divine) within you." It is a Sanskrit word, the sacred language of Hindu scriptures, although the word itself is used more broadly in other faiths and cultures.

The biggest take away I can give you is to stop doing any form of exercise that you hate and makes you feel bad. That's not health. It's not what God or the Universe wants for us. We have such a short time on this beautiful planet of ours. **Don't waste a minute on it moving your body in a way that feels wrong just because you think you're supposed to: "A joyful heart is good medicine, but a crushed spirit dries up the bones." (Proverbs 17:22)**

Find your joyful movement. It's life changing.

Practice Movement and Harmony

Many of us have engaged in certain types of exercise because we felt obligated to do so primarily through diet culture messaging. **When you create space for movement that feels aligned with your soul rather than your fear, you open a doorway to a different kind of connection with your body.** The steps to practice this principle require some experimentation. It is very possible that you may instantly know that some types of movement are not for you. That's okay! Try something else.

Then, after any walk, stretch, yoga session, run, or spontaneous dance break, pause for a moment of reflection. Notice how you felt before you began. Notice how you feel after. Pay attention to any emotional or spiritual shifts. Sometimes movement clears a heavy mood, sometimes it softens stress, and sometimes it simply reminds you that your body is a living, breathing part of creation. If there is a part of you that feels joyful, then lean into that space and dive deeper. It is so cool to find a form of movement that you enjoy doing and that you can slowly improve upon, building mastery and a sense of accomplishment. That said, you do not need to introduce growth goals into your movement routine if by doing so, it becomes a shame-filled obligation. The Universe wants us to find joy. It is not asking for perfection, it is mostly just asking that you show up… preferably in comfortable pants.

Chapter Eleven

Nourish with Love and Wisdom through Gentle Nutrition

During the writing of this book, I am rewatching the iconic series *Golden Girls* with my husband. The first time I watched the series, I was in elementary school. It was the only show my grandmother, my sister, and I could agree on when we would stay with her. I recall really enjoying it, especially the character Rose Nylund. I thought she was hilarious. It is only as I rewatch it as an adult that I realize I only caught about ten percent of the jokes. Now that I catch all the dry humor and endless innuendos, I can fully appreciate this gem of a show. Now that we're watching it again, the character of Sophia Petrillo has become the household favorite. She is feisty, no-nonsense, and has amazing, sarcastic one-liners throughout each episode.

We can infer from some of her classic lines that she would have been in favor of an intuitive eating model. When offered Jell-O, Sophia responded, "If God wanted peaches suspended in mid-air, He'd have filled 'em with helium." We could also infer that in her wisdom, she recognized the risks of dieting. In one episode, she said to her roommate Blanche Devereaux, "The last time you went on a diet, you turned into that guy from *Silence of the Lambs;* you did everything but butter my face." And she loved food. "If this sauce was a person, I'd get naked and make love to it." She loved to cook and would often be seen at the stove stirring her tomato sauce while sharing one of her hilarious stories. To borrow the traditional opening line for all of Sophia's stories, "Picture it: Sicily..."

It's 2011. One of my best friends had invited me to stay with her family in Italy for the summer. It was a dream come true. The entire trip was amazing with so many lifelong memories made. High on that list of memories is the first time I had *pranzo* with her family. *Pranzo,* which means lunch in Sicilian, is the largest meal of the day and typically served in the early afternoon. This was a smorgasbord of the most beautiful mouthwatering food I had ever seen. And it just kept coming—plate after plate of home cooked, made-from-scratch meals served family style. It began with a pasta dish of rigatoni in a rich tomato sauce and fresh basil served with some of the world's best crusty bread. The feast continued with the protein course, either meat or fish, or in my case, *melanzana,* or eggplant. This is seen as a decent substitution here in the States but an exceptional and welcome choice in Sicily. The meal was also typically served with a large, family-style salad and another vegetable or two as sides. Finally, the last course was fresh fruit, which came right from the garden of the home I was staying in. The fruit was juicy and perfect. (Although usually saved for Sundays, I was often treated to a fourth course of dessert because I was spoiled rotten every day of my life-changing trip.)

One of the most important parts of this story, though, is that this experience wasn't happening only in the home I was staying in; this was happening throughout the community, and it still does. Stores close at 1 p.m., and everyone goes home to eat with their family. This idea of taking time to sit down and enjoy a meal with loved ones is in line with what the U.S. Department of Agriculture and the U.S. Department of Health and Human Services describe as eating healthy. The dietary guidelines emphasize meeting nutritional needs through nutrient-dense foods and variety across all food groups as part of a balanced eating pattern. Research associated with the guidelines highlights the importance of shared meals, noting that eating together supports healthy habits, especially in children and families. Leave it to our friendly neighbors to the north to keep it even simpler. Canada's dietary guidelines emphasize eating enough, eating a balanced variety, and eating together.

Across major world religions, food is rarely viewed as morally "good" or "bad" in the way diet culture frames it. Instead, traditions tend to focus on intention, mindfulness, gratitude, community, compassion, and moderation, with food serving as a means of spiritual formation rather than control. In short, they're inherently following many of the intuitive eating guidelines we've already discussed. Further, gentle nutrition encompasses all of this and encourages us to learn about nutrient-dense foods as well as incorporating variety and balance. It invites us to make food choices that care for our bodies and delight our taste buds, marrying nutrition science and internal body wisdom. The focus is on well-being, satisfaction, energy, and kindness over control, guilt, and weight. It advocates for adding nourishing foods in ways that feel supportive and life-giving without turning nutrition into another set of rules and a return to diet culture.

In her beautiful book *Gentle Nutrition: A Non-Diet Approach to Healthy Eating*, Rachael Hartley defines gentle nutrition as "what nutrition looks like when we close our ears to the unscientific and fearmongering babble that makes food out to be the enemy and instead, listen to our body telling us what makes it feel good." She goes on to say that "when nutrition advice aims to shrink bodies, there's an inherent conflict with good nutrition—the kind of nutrition that can actually improve your health."

This is the last principle for a reason. In order to get to the point of gentle nutrition, you've had to push out all of the diet-culture noise and tune in to your body. By doing this, you've laid the foundation of trust necessary for hearing your body speak and allowing it to make the choice of what it needs. That's why making food choices within the intuitive eating model should always be made within the broader context of the first nine principles. If intuitive eating would have asked you to let your body choose before making peace with food or challenging the food police, it would've been pretty hard, maybe even impossible. But you're ready now. Use the wisdom you've learned throughout this journey as your guiding light.

Health Is Not the Only Value

However, even with all of this wisdom, old habits die hard. I can hear that little voice in your head screaming, "But what about eating healthy?! Isn't that important?" You need to kindly tell that little voice to stop being the food police, to simmer down, and to stop yelling at you. Food is fuel. We need it to survive. And yes, there are certainly foods that are more nutritiously-dense than others. Our bodies want and need those nutrients to feel our best. But a prescriptive guide that arbitrarily dictates the same number of servings and the same serving sizes to every person, regardless of age, medical history, gender, and so on isn't "healthy." It can certainly be easier to just follow a prescribed plan, but **feeding one's body is not a one-size-fits-all situation.**

I'm genetically predisposed to high cholesterol, a distance runner, and a vegetarian. In no logical universe should I be telling you to eat how I eat based on my lived experience because my needs are different from yours. Also, and this is important, I'm not a registered dietitian. Nothing creams my corn more than seeing unqualified people providing "expert advice" with no expertise to support it. For example, take your friendly influencer who got all of their followers because of their perfect-looking life with their perfect clothes and perfectly manicured appearance, who then starts trying to convince all five hundred thousand of her followers that in order to be healthy, they need to immediately purge their pantries of everything that has (fill in the blank) ingredient. Combine this with the conspiracy that our food is deliberately poisoning us and the thinking that gaining weight is the ultimate sin, and you have rage bait that will attract thousands of likes and comments because the fear-mongering is compelling and it sells.

It's garbage, my friends. It's unqualified garbage. Go to a cardiologist for a heart issue. Go to a dentist for oral care. Go to a registered dietitian for nutrition advice, and ensure it's a dietitian who is weight inclusive, meaning they focus on health and well-being without promoting weight loss. Unfollow the social media influencers who provide harmful misinformation. While you're at it, don't be afraid to report it in the app. (You can report a comment, the post, or even the account if necessary.) A 2024 study published in the *Psychology of Public Media* found that among university-aged participants who exhibited symptoms of anxiety or depression and who were regular-to-heavy social media users, reducing social media use by about half led to significant improvements in how they felt about their appearance and overall self- esteem. **Take control of your socials and follow accounts that bring you joy, inspiration, and credible education. Where you get your information matters.**

It's also important to consider the role of advertising and marketing in food, specifically on food packaging. You might realize that diet-culture terms like "guilt-free" are clearly marketing terminology, but did you know that "natural" is as well? The term "natural" is not regulated or formally defined by either the Food and Drug Administration (FDA) or the United States Department of Agriculture (USDA). Therefore, it can be inconsistent and misleading. Mix in diet-culture psychology, and we have a whole other problem on our hands. Consider this example. Cookie Box A and Cookie Box B are next to each other on the same shelf, but Cookie Box B says "natural" in lovely bright letters. Without looking at the ingredients, which box of cookies would you think is "healthier"? Before you learned about intuitive eating, which box of cookies would you be most tempted to buy? Yet again clever marketing à la diet culture may persuade us to believe that Cookie Box B is "healthier" despite the higher price. This leads us into the next point about processed foods.

When I share the concept of gentle nutrition, the most common response I receive is the argument around processed foods. "All of this makes sense, Sandi, but it's still not okay to eat a Twinkie." My counter argument: "Why not?" **One snack, one meal, or even one full day of eating less nutrient-dense foods (even if they are ultra-processed and high in sugar like a Twinkie) will not kill you.** Should you eat them every day? No. Should you shame yourself or others for having one? Also, no.

A word about "processed" for a moment. Wow, has this word become weaponized. The truth is that nearly all food is processed to some degree because the simple definition of processed food is any food that has been altered from its original form, typically for the purpose of preservation, safety, convenience, taste, or shelf life. So even more "safe" foods like bagged lettuce, frozen fruits, frozen vegetables, and canned beans are all processed foods—processed and still packed with nutrients.

We typically hear the term "ultra-processed" for more heavily modified alterations including additives, colors, and flavorings. But again, these foods aren't "bad." Food is not an issue of morality. Processed foods can provide easy, efficient, and affordable options with longer shelf lives. No one is saying you should eat this food all the time, but can we please agree to have a kinder tone about this? We all care about health and well-being; however, it's important to remember that everyone's relationship with food is deeply personal. Not everyone has the same access, time, energy, or background when it comes to eating.

This is also part of the challenges of creating a new food pyramid. The USDA first started providing Dietary Guidelines for Americans (DGA) in 1984. Then, every five years, the USDA and the Department of Health and Human Services (HHS) update these guidelines. And how did they choose to communicate this to the general public? The iconic food pyramid. Originally released in 1992, the visual icon conveying the latest recommendations is modified irregularly and not always well-received. After nearly thirteen years, the food pyramid with its horizontally grouped recommendations was replaced with MyPyramid in 2005. This food pyramid was more abstract than the original, changing from six blocks of various sizes to six vertical triangles with physical activity added to the outside of the pyramid. Because of this shift away from clear food-group guidance, people widely criticized it for being abstract and confusing and for requiring online tools to interpret. In response, MyPlate, created in 2011, replaced MyPyramid with a simple plate image that emphasized balance, portion awareness, and practicality.

Then, on January 7th, 2026, the USDA and HHS unveiled the new dietary guidelines, this time in the form of an inverted pyramid. Unsurprisingly, experts have had much discourse and debate on the contents of these new guidelines. The Academy of Nutrition and Dietetics stated "Some of the recommendations in the DGAs (Dietary Guidelines for Americans) are not aligned with the current body of evidence and will create challenges for implementation, particularly across federal nutrition programs that serve millions of Americans." The president of the Academy of Nutrition and Dietetics, Deanne Brandstetter, also noted that "Registered dietitian nutritionists and nutrition and dietetics technicians, registered, play a critical role in applying the DGAs in ways that protect public health and meet the needs of a broad spectrum of populations. However, elements of this version of the guidelines will make that work difficult." This highlights a critical problem with the recommendations themselves. The people creating these policies, tools, and recommendations don't always have the clinical or medical background necessary for interpreting the science, let alone keeping up the latest scientific findings. The food pyramid is constantly critiqued for being overly simplistic, influenced by agricultural and political interests, and for promoting a one-size-fits-all approach to eating. Embedded in that approach is the assumption that everyone has equal access, resources, time, and choice, which we know is not true. This is where the conversation must expand beyond food itself and into the social determinants of health.

We talked about social determinants of health in Chapter 2, a reminder that they are the non-medical but very valid factors that influence our health. If an individual or family is experiencing food insecurity and has very limited resources, then the priority is getting food on the table. All of us should feel free to make food choices that are realistic in terms of access and cost. It is unfair and unkind to judge those who may be living in food deserts, living in poverty, and/or working two jobs to keep food on the table and pay the bills. The last thing needed is judgment for heating up a frozen pizza at the end of a long hard day, ultra-processed or not.

God meets us with kindness and love. Let's try to do the same and trust that loving others is more important than labeling their choices. And that includes your own self-kindness around your own choices and potentially self-imposed rules.

There are some people who take the above arguments very seriously and revolve their lives around eating what they define as "clean" foods. When that level of rigidity is present, it may be an indicator of orthorexia. People with orthorexia often avoid entire food groups, spend excessive time thinking about food quality, and may isolate themselves socially to stick to their eating rules. Although it's not officially recognized as an eating disorder, orthorexia can lead to nutritional problems, mental distress, and a poor quality of life. Those with orthorexia may experience extreme guilt or anxiety around eating non "pure" foods and feel a sense of superiority when adhering to the "safe foods." People with orthorexia see "clean" eating as part of their identity. The fixation and preoccupation can take over their lives but because it's disguised as health behaviors, it is often difficult to shift the perspective for these individuals to see the way it is creating an unhealthy lifestyle.

This also feels like a good time to address the counterargument I hear at times in regards to "the body is a temple," which is a passage very often taken out of context. This passage originated in the Bible in the book of Corinthians and was used to convey that the body is a dwelling place for the Holy Spirit, and therefore, must be treated with care and respect. And, yes! As we discussed at length in Chapter 9: Respect Your Body, we absolutely should take care of it. It's the only one we'll ever have. But this phrase has been twisted and weaponized into shaming people about ingesting any food that isn't considered "clean." Let that go. You can feel confident that you are treating your body like a temple if you aren't hurting it by ignoring your hunger or fullness and instead listening intuitively to God's beautiful design. **Across faith traditions, the spiritual concern is rarely about controlling the body. Instead, food is a sacred means of connection to God, to community, to the earth, and to oneself.** Food hierarchies for the sake of appearance, punishment, or moral superiority are noticeably absent. What matters is intention, care, balance, gratitude, and compassion.

For example, across many Indigenous cultures, food is understood as a sacred gift from the Creator, not a commodity and not a moral test. Eating is not simply about fueling a body but about participating in a relationship that has existed long before us and will continue after us. In these traditions, the body is not something to conquer or control. It is part of creation itself. No one's worth is measured by how they eat or what their body looks like.

The emphasis is on making sure everyone is fed, honored, and included. This directly challenges diet culture, which thrives on separation, comparison, and scarcity.

Even if you're not quite ready to throw out all the rules and listen intuitively, and believe me that can definitely take time, I hope you will remember that while health is important, it's not the only thing that's important. There are so many more values to live by: Courage. Empathy. Honesty. Kindness. Humility. Accountability. Curiosity. Resiliency. Generosity. Compassion. Integrity. Love. Gratitude. Tolerance, Friendship. Loyalty. Trustworthiness. Joy. Connection. Faith.

These are twenty of probably a hundred different values that we could name. Depending on the situation, each of these can be considered just as important as health, and in some cases, even more important. Health matters, but it is not the only value that matters.

Ask yourself this question: Would you be willing to live five extra years if you knew those years would be riddled with loneliness, depression, and misery? I'm guessing probably not. And if I'm right, it tells me you recognize (even if it's deep down) that joy and connections make life worth living.

Therefore, feed your body with gentle nutrition. Provide it the fuel and pleasure you need and deserve. But please, don't limit yourself to believing that this is all that matters. We will all get sick, and we will all eventually succumb to the inevitably of death. I believe that so much of what drives our insistence and obsession with being "healthy" is driven by death anxiety, a Freudian and psychoanalytical therapy concept. Being rigid about food choices (for example, not having the slice of birthday cake) is a subconscious effort at trying to have more control over our own inevitable demise. But this is an illusion. *Buddha's Little Instruction Book* reminds us, "The trouble is, you think you have time." Therefore, I refuse to allow each remaining day I have to be about "trying to get healthy" instead of living a full, holistically healthy approach to life that encompasses my body, yes, but equally as important, also encompasses my mental and spiritual health.

So eat the kale salad if you like kale! Especially the one with olive oil, lemon, garlic, and parmesan (so good!). *And* eat the birthday cake with buttercream icing. But above all else, be gentle with yourself.

A Lifetime of Enjoyment

The co-founders of intuitive eating, Tribole and Resch, define gentle nutrition as "making food choices that honor your well-being, taste buds, and culture, while attuning to how your body feels." They go on to say that you don't have to eat perfectly to be healthy, and you won't suddenly get a nutrient deficiency from one snack, one meal, or one day of eating. What you eat consistently over time is what matters, as your food choices and movement only account for about ten percent of your health.

To this point, all clinicians in this space would agree on the idea of additions versus subtractions. In other words, **it's not about taking specific foods or groups of foods out like diet culture does. It's about adding foods in.** Here's an example: Your favorite snack is potato chips. Most diets would tell you to cut those out. But as we've learned in the last ten chapters, diets don't work. So instead of eliminating a snack that brings you satisfaction and pleasure, ask yourself, "What can I add?" Perhaps that means having a variety of snacks available to you in the home, including your beloved chips. It could look like snacking on some chips to honor that hunger but switching to something else when that need has been satisfied. If you're still hungry, eat something like cheese and crackers, Greek yogurt with berries, or apples with peanut butter. It may take some time to find what feels best. Progress, not perfection, is what counts.

I love this so much. You finally get to the last principle, and there still isn't a section on "you must eat X amount of this" or "Y grams of that" or "Z combination of macros" because there is no secret, mysterious, magical one-size-fits-all plan. Yes, you should aim for nutrient dense foods. Yes, you should eat your fruits and veggies. As God said, "Behold, I have given you every plant yielding seed that is on the face of all the earth, and every tree with seed in its fruit. You shall have them for food." (Genesis 1:29) Yes, protein-rich foods and quality fats are also important. And yes, you should have a variety of foods from different food groups. Tribole and Resch specifically mention eating *enough* fruits, vegetables, and grains, and drinking enough water. But that's really as specific as it gets!

Gentle nutrition provides a beautiful model, but it can be somewhat challenging at first. It's important to remember that gentle nutrition is intentionally open. The founders stayed true to their first nine principles by not being prescriptive or providing any one-size-fits-all meal plan in principle ten. **We each have a unique biology and lifestyle and therefore need unique and individualized meal plans.** If you're still feeling a bit frustrated with not having a clear set of rules, I get it. We have been inundated with various rules about how to eat and what to eat and when to eat for forever, so the absence of that can feel confusing and a bit daunting. But there is also freedom in that. Freedom to listen intuitively to your body's needs.

In the Hindu tradition, the practice of offering *prasad* teaches that food is sacred and a gift to be prepared and received with gratitude and awareness. *Prasad* literally means grace or divine gift. Food is given as an offering during worship, it is blessed, and then shared with the community. It is a sacred exchange between humans and the divine and turns simple food into a spiritual experience. This mirrors the principle of gentle nutrition beautifully and invites us to nourish our bodies with care rather than control. Although nutrients matter, no food is inherently good or bad; each food can serve a purpose, including physical, emotional, and, yes, spiritual. When we approach eating with reverence instead of judgment, every meal becomes a chance to honor both the body and the divine. In this way, choosing and sharing food becomes not just an act of nourishment, but an act of love and connection.

Gentle nutrition offers a way to care for health without fear, perfectionism, or shame. Instead of demanding rigid rules or "fixing" the body, it meets people where they are and builds nourishment on a foundation of self-trust, compassion, and realism. That alone is profoundly regulating for the nervous system and especially healing for anyone who has been harmed by diet culture and moralized food advice. Gentle nutrition recognizes that nutrients matter, and so do access, culture, pleasure, energy levels, mental health, trauma history, finances, and time. It invites curiosity instead of compliance. Rather than asking, "Am I doing this right?" it asks "How does this feel in my body?" By following the path of gentle nutrition, you enter into a hopeful relationship with food where trust replaces tension and nourishment becomes a quiet practice of devotion.

Practice Gentle Nutrition

When you begin to view your health choices as acts of reverence rather than restriction, something inside you may soften. It becomes less about following rules and more about caring for the body that carries you through this life. From this perspective, feeding yourself is no longer a battleground. It becomes a quiet practice of love. Consider journaling or talking to someone you trust about your personal values. What happens when you prioritize values in addition to the value of health? For example, what would it look like to set goals around values such as bravery, generosity, friendship, and devotion rather than trying to eat perfectly?

You might find that good food helps you show up with more clarity, presence, patience, and joy. As you explore this connection, choose one small, compassionate nutrition habit that feels supportive. It should feel like a gift, not a punishment. Food becomes less about taking things away and more about adding what supports your energy, stability, grounding, and spiritual clarity. Gentle nutrition thrives on addition. It is far more powerful to ask, "What can I add that will help me feel more alive, more supported, more connected?" rather than, "What should I eliminate?" When you focus on adding, there is less fear and more abundance. Your meals become places where kindness shows up on the plate.

Practice choosing meals based on genuine satisfaction and how you want to feel afterward. Notice the foods that help you feel energized, stable, grounded, or even spiritually connected.

These subtle shifts are not about perfection. They are about honoring yourself in small, steady ways. Gentle nutrition becomes a kind of prayer, a way of saying "I am worthy of care, comfort, and nourishment." Every choice is an invitation to care for yourself with a little more tenderness than before. And if embracing that feels like a small miracle, that is because it is.

Conclusion

We've been through a lot together. I suspect this may have felt like an emotional roller coaster. Here's the thing: You have total control over your next steps. Perhaps this book has felt as if it was speaking to you directly, and you feel motivated and ready to throw out the diet books and the scale and start practicing the principles we've discussed today. Or perhaps you still have questions and want to connect with an intuitive eating clinician to discuss your personal journey. As the American author Annie Dillard writes, "How we spend our days is, of course, how we spend our lives." Let that sink in. **This is an opportunity to stand up against the oppression that is diet culture and replace it with what really matters: your most earnest hopes and values.**

Above all else, my sincere prayer is that this book has helped you feel less alone. I hope it has helped provide you with a bit more direction or at least things to reflect on going forward. But if there are those of you who are having some big feelings and are a bit confused on where to start, remember that God really only put one thing on our must-do list: "Love others as I have loved you."

For me, that is a crystal-clear blueprint for how to guide my thoughts, actions, and decisions. That is the path. I ask myself on a daily basis, "Is the way I am spending my time, energy, and resources leading with love?" In the absence of all the noise in my brain since I told diet culture to get lost, I try to fill my brain back up with that thought and my connection to my faith and others, guided by love and kindness.

No matter where you are in your journey, I am so proud of you. I sincerely hope you feel proud of yourself. It is a radical act to decide to love yourself as you are and not how others would have us be. It is a courageous act to make big changes at any stage of life in the pursuit of faith, joy, and connection.

Bob Goff poignantly writes, "Here's a truth you can take to the bank no matter how long you live: The clarity of purpose, undistracted energy, selfless love, and unselfish pursuits you bring to the world will be your legacy. Everything else will look like a distraction by comparison." **You were always made for more. You are a child of the great divine. You are a masterpiece.** You are special and unique and loved. The shape of your body does not define you. Your weight is not your worth. You have so much to give, and you deserve to be happy TODAY. No longer will you allow others to tell you that you aren't good enough exactly as you are. You have the choice to not spend another moment or another dollar on thoughts and things that are trying to "fix" you when you are not broken.

Take a deep breath, my friend. Be brave. Let the nonsense go. Grab on tight to what really matters. Love. Joy. Faith. Connection. We don't have as much time as we think we do, and you are not alone. There is an ever-growing community of people who are following this path. My sincerest hope is that you continue on this journey. It has been life-changing for me and for countless others. I can't wait for you to be part of it.

And I hope you begin to see yourself as God and the Universe see you. Because you, my friend, are extraordinary. The light within me honors the light within you. *Namaste.*

My beloved child,
break your heart no longer.
Each time you judge yourself
you break your own heart.

You stop feeding on the love,
which is the wellspring of your vitality.
The time has come, your time
To live, to celebrate…
and to see the goodness that you are…

Let no one, no thing, no idea or ideal obstruct you
If one comes, even in the name of "Truth",
forgive it for its unknowing

Do not fight
Let go
And breathe — into the goodness that you are.

—Swami Kripaluanandaji (Bapuji)

Resources and Support

Books

Alissa Rumsey, *Unapologetic Eating*, 2021

Anna Yusim, *Fulfilled*, 2017

Aubrey Gordon, Y*ou Just Need to Lose Weight*, 2023

Aubrey Gordon, *What We Don't Talk about When We Talk About Fat*, 2020

Bob Goff, *Undistracted*, 2022.

Christy Harrison, *Anti-Diet*, 2019

Evelyn Tribole and Elyse Resch, *Intuitive Eating 4th Ed*, 2020

Evelyn Tribole and Elyse Resch, *The Intuitive Eating Workbook*, 2025

Gretchen Rubin, *Secrets of Adulthood*, 2025

Lexie and Lindsay Kite, *More Than a Body*, 2020

Lindo Bacon, *Body Respect*, 2014

Lindo Bacon, *Health at Every Size: The Surprising Truth About Your Weight*, 2010

Rachael Hartley, *Gentle Nutrition*, 2021

Sabring Strings, *Fearing the Black Body*, 2019

Shana Minei Spence, *Live Nourished*, 2024

Sonya Renee Taylor, *The Body is Not an Apology*, 2018

Summer Brooks and Amee Severson, *How to Raise and Intuitive Eater*, 2022

Support*

Find a therapist at www.psychologytoday.com

Find a dietician at www.eatright.org/find-a-nutrition-expert

*Look for words in bios like *anti-diet, weight inclusive,* and *HAES aligned*

Research and Sources

Andersen, A. E. 2022. "Diagnosis and Treatment of the Eating Disorder Spectrum in Primary Care Medicine." In *Eating Disorders: A Comprehensive Guide to Medical Care and Complications*, 4th ed., edited by P. S. Mehler and A. E. Andersen, 1–106. Johns Hopkins University Press. https://doi.org/10.1007/s40519-022-01479-3.

Bacon, Linda, and Lucy Aphramor. 2011. "Weight Science: Evaluating the Evidence for a Paradigm Shift." *Nutrition Journal* 10 (9): 1–13.

Batorek, M., and I. Hromatko. 2024. "Cognitive Functions, Mood and Sleep Quality after Two Months of Intermittent Fasting." *Journal of Trial and Error* 1. https://doi.org/10.36850/e71f-5cff.

Brooks, Sumner, and Amee Severson. 2022. *How to Raise an Intuitive Eater: Raising the Next Generation with Food and Body Confidence.* St. Martin's Essentials.

Centers for Disease Control and Prevention. 2011. "Diabetes in Youth: United States, 2001–2009." *Morbidity and Mortality Weekly Report* 60 (5): 1–23.

Dietitians of Canada. 2019. "Unlocking the Potential of Food: A Healthy Eating Pattern for Canadians." In *Canada's Dietary Guidelines*, 10–30. Health Canada.

Fothergill, Eric, Juen Guo, Lori Howard, Jennifer C. Kerns, Naji D. Knuth, Robert Brychta, Kong Y. Chen, et al. 2016. "Persistent Metabolic Adaptation 6 Years after 'The Biggest Loser' Competition." *Obesity* 24 (8): 1612–1619. https://doi.org/10.1002/oby.21538.

Gilbert, Elizabeth. 2015. *Big Magic: Creative Living beyond Fear.* Riverhead Books.

Hartley, Rachael. 2021. *Gentle Nutrition: A Non-Diet Approach to Healthy Eating.* Victory Belt Publishing.

Jansen, Esther L. G. M., Sandra Mulkens, and Anita T. M. Jansen. 2007. "Do Not Eat the Red Food! Prohibition of Snacks Leads to Their Relatively Higher Consumption in Children." *Appetite* 49 (3): 572–577.

Kaiser Family Foundation. 2024. "Poll: One in Eight Adults Say They've Taken a GLP-1 Drug, Including 4 in 10 of Those with Diabetes and 1 in 4 of Those with Heart Disease." *KFF Health Tracking Poll,* May 10.

Kolata, Gina. 2016. "After 'The Biggest Loser,' Their Bodies Fought to Regain Weight." *New York Times*, May 2. https://www.nytimes.com/2016/05/02/health/biggest-loser-weight-loss.html.

Latner, Janet D., Kerry S. O'Brien, Lori E. Durso, Willem P. Brinkman, and Tracy MacDonald. 2008. "Weighing Obesity Stigma: The Relative Strength of Different Forms of Bias." *International Journal of Obesity* 32 (7): 1145–1152.

Linardon, Jake, and Tracy L. Tylka. 2018. "Associations between Intuitive Eating and Health Indicators: A Systematic Review of Observational and Intervention Studies." *Appetite* 123: 50–59. https://doi.org/10.1016/j.appet.2017.11.016.

Mann, Traci, A. Janet Tomiyama, Erica Westling, Anne-Marie Lew, and B. Samuels. 2007. "Medicare's Search for Effective Obesity Treatments: Diets Are Not the Answer." *American Psychologist* 62 (3): 220–233.

Mayer-Davis, Elizabeth J., Dana Dabelea, Jean M. Lawrence, et al. 2021. "Trends in Prevalence of Type 1 and Type 2 Diabetes in

Children and Adolescents in the U.S., 2001–2017." *JAMA* 326 (8): 717–727. https://doi.org/10.1001/jama.2021.11165.

Medical Students for Size Inclusivity. 2023. *GLP-1 Agonist Medications: Informed Consent Resource.* November. https://sizeinclusivemedicine.org/glp1/.

Menniti, G., S. Meshkat, Q. Lin, W. Lou, A. Reichelt, and V. Bhat. 2025. "Mental Health Consequences of Dietary Restriction: Increased Depressive Symptoms in Biological Men and Populations with Elevated BMI." *BMJ Nutrition, Prevention & Health* 8 (1): e001167.

Naous, Elie, Ahmad Achkar, and Joyce Mitri. 2023. "Intermittent Fasting and Its Effects on Weight, Glycemia, Lipids, and Blood Pressure: A Narrative Review." *Nutrients* 15 (16): 3661. https://doi.org/10.3390/nu15163661.

National Health and Medical Research Council. 2013. *Clinical Practice Guidelines for the Management of Overweight and Obesity in Adults, Adolescents and Children in Australia.* https://www.nhmrc.gov.au/about-us/publications/clinical-practice-guidelines-management-overweight-and-obesity.

Péneau, Sandrine, Estelle Ménard, Caroline Méjean, France Bellisle, and Serge Hercberg. 2013. "Sex and Dieting Modify the Association between Emotional Eating and Weight Status." *American Journal of Clinical Nutrition* 97 (6): 1307–1313. https://doi.org/10.3945/ajcn.112.054916.

Puhl, Rebecca, and Chelsea Heuer. 2010. "Obesity Stigma: Important Considerations for Public Health." *American Journal of Public Health* 100 (6): 1019–1028. https://doi.org/10.2105/AJPH.2009.159491.

Puhl, Rebecca, Janna Luedicke, and Chelsea Heuer. 2011. "Weight-Based Victimization toward Overweight Adolescents:

Observations and Reactions of Peers." *Journal of School Health* 81 (12): 696–703.

Puhl, Rebecca, Janna Luedicke, and Chelsea Heuer. 2024. "Fad Dieting and Psychological Well-Being: Associations with Depression and Body Shame." *Eating Behaviors.*

Puhl, Rebecca M., and Y. Suh. 2015. "Health Consequences of Weight Stigma: Implications for Obesity Prevention and Treatment." *Current Obesity Reports* 4 (2): 182–190. https://doi.org/10.1007/s13679-015-0153-z.

Rozzell, Katherine, Daniel Y. Moon, Paul Klimek, Taylor Brown, and Aaron J. Blashill. 2019. "Prevalence of Eating Disorders among U.S. Children Aged 9 to 10 Years: Data from the Adolescent Brain Cognitive Development Study." *JAMA Pediatrics* 173 (1): 100–101.

Rubin, Gretchen. 2009. *The Happiness Project.* HarperCollins.

Rubin, Gretchen. 2025. *Secrets of Adulthood: Simple Truths for Our Complex Lives.* Crown.

Solmi, Francesca, Karin W. Hagberg, Christina Dalman, Robin M. Gardner, and Joseph F. Hayes. 2022. "Age at Onset of Mental Disorders: A Meta-Analysis of Population-Based Studies." *JAMA Psychiatry* 79 (5): 447–456.

Stunkard, Albert J., James R. Harris, Nancy L. Pedersen, and Gerald E. McClearn. 1990. "The Body-Mass Index of Twins Who Have Been Reared Apart." *New England Journal of Medicine* 322 (21): 1483–1487.

Swartz, Amanda Z., K. Wood, E. Farber-Eger, A. Petty, and Heidi J. Silver. 2025. "Weight Trajectory Impacts Risk for 10 Distinct Cardiometabolic Diseases." *Journal of Clinical Endocrinology*

& Metabolism. Advance online publication. https://doi.org/10.1210/clinem/dgaf348.

Thai, H., C. G. Davis, W. Mahboob, S. Perry, A. Adams, and G. S. Goldfield. 2024. "Reducing Social Media Use Improves Appearance and Weight Esteem in Youth with Emotional Distress." *Psychology of Popular Media* 13 (1): 162–169. https://doi.org/10.1037/ppm000046.

Tomiyama, A. Janet, Jeffrey M. Hunger, Julia Nguyen-Cuu, and Christie Wells. 2016. "Misclassification of Cardiometabolic Health When Using Body Mass Index Categories in NHANES 2005–2012." *International Journal of Obesity* 40 (5): 883–886. https://doi.org/10.1038/ijo.2016.17.

The Trevor Project. 2022. *2022 National Survey on LGBTQ Youth Mental Health.* December 15. https://www.thetrevorproject.org/survey-2022/.

Tribole, Evelyn, and Elyse Resch. 2020. *Intuitive Eating: A Revolutionary Anti-Diet Approach.* 4th ed. St. Martin's Essentials.

Tribole, Evelyn, and Elyse Resch. 2025. *The Intuitive Eating Workbook: Ten Principles for Nourishing a Healthy Relationship with Food.* 2nd ed. New Harbinger Publications.

U.S. Department of Agriculture and U.S. Department of Health and Human Services. 2020. *Dietary Guidelines for Americans, 2020–2025.* 9th ed. https://www.dietaryguidelines.gov/.

Wang, H., W. He, G. Yang, L. Zhu, and X. Liu. 2024. "The Impact of Weight Cycling on Health and Obesity." *Metabolites* 14 (6): 344.

Weight Watchers International, Inc. 2001. *Annual Report 2001.* U.S. Securities and Exchange Commission.

Wildman, Rachel P., Paul Muntner, Kristi Reynolds, Aidan P. McGinn, Saurabh Rajpathak, Judith Wylie-Rosett, and Mary R. Sowers. 2008. "The Obese without Cardiometabolic Risk Factor Clustering and the Normal Weight with Cardiometabolic Risk Factor Clustering." *Archives of Internal Medicine* 168 (15): 1617–1624. https://doi.org/10.1001/archinte.168.15.1617.

Wu, Y. K., and Diane C. Berry. 2018. "Impact of Weight Stigma on Physiological and Psychological Health Outcomes for Overweight and Obese Adults: A Systematic Review." *Journal of Advanced Nursing* 74 (5): 1030–1042. https://doi.org/10.1111/jan.13511.

YouGov. 2020. "Which Diet Works Best?" February 19. https://today.yougov.com/consumer/articles/28065-most-effective-diet-intermittent-fasting-poll.

Yusim, Anna. 2017. *Fulfilled: How the Science of Spirituality Can Help You Live a Happier, More Meaningful Life*. Grand Central Life & Style.

Zhao, Y., and William Encinosa. 2009. *Hospitalizations for Eating Disorders from 1999 to 2006.* HCUP Statistical Brief No. 70. Agency for Healthcare Research and Quality.

Zhong, F., T. Zhu, X. Jin, X. Chen, R. Wu, L. Shao, and S. Wang. 2024. "Adverse Events Profile Associated with Intermittent Fasting in Adults with Overweight or Obesity: A Systematic Review and Meta-Analysis of Randomized Controlled Trials." *Nutrition Journal* 23: 72. https://doi.org/10.1186/s12937-024-00975-9.

Websites

Association for Size Diversity and Health: HAES Principles
asdah.org/haes

Feed Your Purpose
www.feedyourpurposebook.com

Intuitive Eating: The Original Intuitive Eating Pros
www.intuitiveeating.org

International Association of Eating Disorder Professionals
iaedpfoundation.com

National Eating Disorder Association
www.nationaleatingdisorders.org

National Association of Anorexia and Associated Disorders
anad.org

National Alliance for Eating Disorders
www.allianceforeatingdisorders.com

Acknowledgments

This book would not be possible without the courage and honesty of those who have shared their truths with me over the years about the pain and years lost due to diet culture, disordered eating, eating disorders, and decades of hating their bodies. I have a more complete sense of systemic failures of diet culture because of you.

This book stands on the shoulders of the many clinicians and activists fighting against diet culture and weight stigma. You are each an inspiration. This book would not exist without the dedication and innovation of Evelyn Tribole and Elyse Resch, who first developed intuitive eating and have changed countless lives as a result, including mine.

I had the pleasure and honor of meeting with many different individuals and spiritual leaders across different faiths and traditions for background on this book. Thank you for your honesty, your authenticity and the work you do every day in service of others.

I am so grateful to have found an editor who understood and shared my vision for this book from our first conversation. Thank you, Erin Harris, for seeing its potential.

As a person with minimal visual art skills, I am so grateful to have had such a talented artist in Andrea Boucher to work with on the cover design, formatting and copy edits.

I am indebted to my social work training and social work community. I have had many titles in various positions across my career, but I have always been and will always be proud of being a social worker. The values of social justice and equal rights for all fuels me every day.

I am always and forever grateful to the public library system for not only providing me a quiet space to research and write, but for all of the work they do for communities every day.

I have been so fortunate to have a network of friends who are therapists and dieticians in this space. They are amazing and strong and so incredibly smart. I feel fortunate to be in their circle.

Although terrified, I allowed six people to read the first draft of my book. Thank you for your honest feedback and for your love for me and this project.

I would not be the person I am today without my loving parents, my wonderful sisters, and my incredible extended family all over the country. And especially my mom, who told me I was "brilliant" more times than I can count for my entire life. I'm where I am because I believed you.

I have been so blessed with the women in my life. I have so many girlfriends who are ride-or-die, and I am very aware of how lucky I am to know I can call any of you at any time and you will be there for me.

There's no one on this planet like my husband Andrew. You are the perfect man and partner and I adore you. Thank you for loving me and believing in me.

For my pack waiting for me at the rainbow bridge, Mama loves you.

About the Author

Sandi Morse is a licensed therapist and intuitive eating counselor who writes at the intersection of nutrition, mental health, and spirituality. Drawing on decades of clinical experience, she helps people untangle from diet culture and rediscover the wisdom of the body. She lives in Texas with her husband and their velociraptor (six-month-old puppy) Gus Gus.

www.ingramcontent.com/pod-product-compliance
Lightning Source LLC
LaVergne TN
LVHW090400210926
848480LV00002B/405